The Pregnancy Blueprint: Navigating the Path to Parenthood

Elena Olivera

Table of Contents

Introduction

Chapter 1: Discovering the News

The First Signs

Discovering that you are pregnant can be one of the most exhilarating, surprising, and life-changing moments of your life. It often begins with a few subtle signs that your body is undergoing significant changes. The earliest symptoms of pregnancy vary widely but can include missed periods, tender or swollen breasts, nausea (often referred to as morning sickness), increased urination, and fatigue. These symptoms, while common in early pregnancy, can also be mistaken for other conditions or stressors, so they may not immediately signal pregnancy to every woman.

For many, the realization starts with a missed period, especially if they have regular menstrual cycles. This can prompt a sense of curiosity or anxiety, leading to the next step: confirming the pregnancy with a test.

Taking a Home Pregnancy Test

Home pregnancy tests are widely available, affordable, and straightforward to use, making them the first go-to method for confirming pregnancy. These tests work by detecting the presence of human chorionic gonadotropin (hCG), a hormone produced by the placenta shortly after the embryo attaches to the uterine lining. Most home pregnancy tests claim to be 99% accurate when used correctly, and many can detect pregnancy as early as the first day of a missed period.

When taking a home pregnancy test, it's essential to follow the instructions carefully to ensure accurate results. Typically, the test involves dipping a test strip into a urine sample or placing the strip in the stream of urine. The results usually appear within a few minutes, with a positive test showing two lines or a plus sign, and a negative test showing one line or a minus sign.

Despite the reliability of home pregnancy tests, false negatives can occur, especially if the test is taken too early, when hCG levels are still low. Therefore, if you suspect you are pregnant but receive a negative result, it's advisable to wait a few days and retest or consult a healthcare provider for a more definitive test.

Confirming with a Doctor

Once you have a positive home pregnancy test, the next step is to confirm the pregnancy with a healthcare provider. This typically involves a blood test, which can measure the exact levels of hCG and provide a more accurate confirmation of pregnancy. Your doctor may also perform a physical examination and an ultrasound to confirm the pregnancy and estimate its gestational age.

During your first prenatal visit, your healthcare provider will gather your medical history, conduct a physical exam, and discuss any symptoms you may be experiencing. This is also an opportunity to ask questions and receive guidance on how to care for yourself and your developing baby throughout the pregnancy.

The Emotional Rollercoaster

Discovering that you are pregnant can trigger a whirlwind of emotions. For some, it's a moment of sheer joy and excitement, especially if the pregnancy was planned and eagerly anticipated. For others, the news may come as a surprise, leading to mixed emotions, including fear, anxiety, and uncertainty. It's normal to feel a range of emotions, and every reaction is valid.

Expectant mothers often feel a sense of awe and wonder at the realization that a new life is growing inside them. This can be accompanied by a strong sense of responsibility and a desire to do everything possible to ensure a healthy pregnancy. At the same time, it's also common to feel overwhelmed by the changes ahead and the unknowns that come with parenthood.

Coping with the News

Coping with the discovery of pregnancy involves not only managing physical symptoms but also addressing the emotional and psychological impact of this significant life event. It's important to give yourself time to process the news and to seek support from loved ones, whether it's your partner, family, or friends. Sharing your feelings and concerns can help alleviate some of the anxiety and provide a sense of comfort and reassurance.

If the pregnancy was unplanned, it's especially important to take time to consider your options and what feels right for you. This might include seeking counseling or talking to a healthcare provider to explore all available options and make an informed decision.

Informing Your Partner and Loved Ones

Telling your partner and loved ones about the pregnancy is another significant step. How and when to share the news is a personal decision and can depend on various factors, including your relationship dynamics, timing, and personal preferences.

Some may choose to share the news with their partner immediately, wanting to involve them from the very beginning. Others might wait until they have confirmed the pregnancy with a healthcare provider or until they feel more emotionally prepared to share the news.

When it comes to informing family and friends, some couples prefer to wait until the end of the first trimester, when the risk of miscarriage significantly decreases. Others may choose to share the news earlier, especially if they feel they need additional support.

Planning for the Future

Once the initial excitement and emotions settle, practical considerations come into play. Pregnancy is a time of planning and preparation, not just for the arrival of the baby but also for the many changes that will occur in your life. This includes planning for prenatal care, adjusting your lifestyle to support a healthy pregnancy, and preparing for the financial, emotional, and logistical aspects of bringing a new life into the world.

Prenatal Care and Health

Ensuring you receive proper prenatal care is crucial for the health of both you and your baby. This involves regular check-ups with your healthcare provider, where they will monitor the progress of your pregnancy, perform necessary tests, and provide guidance on nutrition, exercise, and overall well-being.

During your prenatal visits, your doctor will track your baby's growth, check for any potential complications, and offer advice on managing pregnancy symptoms. They will also discuss important milestones, such as prenatal screening tests, ultrasounds, and the timeline for major prenatal care events.

Nutrition and Lifestyle Adjustments

A healthy diet and lifestyle are vital for a successful pregnancy. This includes eating a balanced diet rich in essential nutrients, such as folic acid, iron, calcium, and omega-3 fatty acids, which support the development of your baby and maintain your own health. Avoiding harmful substances, such as alcohol, tobacco, and certain medications, is also critical.

Exercise is another important aspect of a healthy pregnancy. Engaging in regular, moderate physical activity can help manage weight, reduce stress, and prepare your body for labor and delivery. However, it's important to consult with your healthcare provider before starting any new exercise regimen.

Emotional and Psychological Well-being

Maintaining your emotional and psychological well-being is just as important as your physical health during pregnancy. Hormonal changes, physical discomfort, and the anticipation of parenthood can all contribute to fluctuating emotions. Practicing self-care, engaging in relaxation techniques, and seeking support from loved ones can help manage stress and promote a positive pregnancy experience.

Financial Planning

Pregnancy and childbirth can bring significant financial responsibilities. It's important to plan for the costs associated with prenatal care, delivery, and baby essentials. This might include reviewing your health insurance coverage, creating a budget, and starting a savings plan to cover additional expenses.

Preparing Your Home

Preparing your home for the arrival of a new baby is another key aspect of the journey. This involves setting up a nursery, ensuring you have all the necessary baby supplies, and baby-proofing your home to create a safe environment. It's also helpful to plan for any changes in your living arrangements or routines that will accommodate the new addition to your family.

Reflecting on the Journey

As you embark on the journey of pregnancy, it's important to take time to reflect on the experience and appreciate the incredible transformation your body and life are undergoing. Every pregnancy is unique, and embracing the journey with an open heart and mind can make the experience more rewarding.

Emotions:

Initial Reactions

Discovering that you are pregnant can elicit a wide array of emotions, each unique to the individual and their circumstances. The initial reaction often hinges on whether the pregnancy was planned, a delightful surprise, or an unexpected shock. For many, a positive pregnancy test brings overwhelming joy and excitement, particularly if they've been eagerly anticipating this moment. The thought of bringing a new life into the world can fill you with a sense of wonder and profound happiness.

However, if the pregnancy is unexpected, the initial response might be more complex. Feelings of shock, disbelief, and anxiety are common. You might find yourself grappling with a sense of uncertainty about the future and the immense responsibility that comes with parenthood. It's essential to remember that these feelings are entirely normal and that it's okay to take time to process the news.

Joy and Excitement

For those who have been trying to conceive, discovering a pregnancy can be a dream come true. The excitement of starting a new chapter, the joy of creating a family, and the anticipation of meeting your baby can be overwhelmingly positive. This joy often motivates expectant mothers to immediately begin planning and preparing for the baby's arrival, from decorating the nursery to selecting names.

This period can also bring a deep sense of connection with your partner, as you share the joy and responsibilities of expecting a child. Celebrating this news together can strengthen your bond and lay the foundation for a supportive and loving parenting partnership.

Anxiety and Fear

Regardless of how desired a pregnancy is, it is natural to experience anxiety and fear. Concerns about the baby's health, the potential for complications, and the life changes that lie ahead can weigh heavily on your mind. The physical changes and symptoms of pregnancy can also contribute to feelings of apprehension.

Financial worries are another common source of anxiety. The cost of prenatal care, delivery, and raising a child can be daunting, especially if you feel unprepared financially. Creating a budget and planning for these expenses can help mitigate some of these concerns.

Uncertainty and Doubt

If the pregnancy was not planned, or if there are challenging circumstances surrounding it, you might experience a significant amount of uncertainty and doubt. Questions about your readiness to become a parent, your ability to provide for the child, and how this change will affect your career, relationships, and lifestyle can be overwhelming.

It's important to give yourself permission to feel these emotions without judgment. Seeking advice from trusted friends, family members, or a counselor can provide perspective and support as you navigate these uncertainties.

Mixed Emotions

It's also common to experience a blend of emotions simultaneously. You might feel elated and anxious, joyful and fearful, excited and uncertain—all at the same time. Pregnancy is a major life transition, and mixed emotions are a natural part of this journey. Allow yourself to feel these emotions and acknowledge that they are a normal response to a significant change.

Managing Emotional Health

Maintaining emotional health during pregnancy is crucial for both your well-being and that of your baby. Here are some strategies to help you cope with the emotional rollercoaster of discovering you are pregnant:

1. **Communicate Your Feelings:**
   - Sharing your emotions with your partner, family, or close friends can provide relief and support. Open communication helps to process your feelings and can strengthen your relationships.
2. **Seek Support:**
   - Joining a prenatal support group or engaging in online forums can connect you with other expectant mothers who are experiencing similar emotions. These communities can offer valuable advice, empathy, and encouragement.
3. **Practice Self-Care:**
   - Prioritize activities that promote relaxation and well-being. This could include taking gentle walks, practicing yoga or meditation, reading, or engaging in hobbies that bring you joy.
4. **Educate Yourself:**
   - Learning about pregnancy, childbirth, and parenting can reduce anxiety by making you feel more prepared and informed. Attend prenatal classes, read books, and consult reliable sources for information.

5. **Professional Help:**
   - If you find that your emotions are overwhelming or if you are experiencing signs of depression or severe anxiety, consider seeking help from a mental health professional. Prenatal counselors and therapists can provide support and coping strategies.
6. **Maintain a Healthy Lifestyle:**
   - Eating a balanced diet, getting regular exercise, and ensuring adequate rest can positively impact your emotional well-being. Physical health and mental health are closely linked, and taking care of your body can help stabilize your emotions.
7. **Mindfulness and Relaxation Techniques:**
   - Techniques such as deep breathing exercises, progressive muscle relaxation, and mindfulness meditation can help manage stress and anxiety. These practices can be integrated into your daily routine to provide ongoing emotional support.

Long-term Emotional Preparation

As you move beyond the initial discovery phase, your emotions will continue to evolve. It's helpful to remain mindful of your emotional state and to regularly check in with yourself about how you're feeling. Preparing emotionally for the changes that parenthood will bring involves:

- **Setting Realistic Expectations:**
  - Understand that it's normal to have good days and bad days. Pregnancy and parenthood are not always picture-perfect, and it's okay to have moments of doubt or difficulty.
- **Building a Support Network:**
  - Cultivate relationships with people who can offer practical and emotional support. This network might include your partner, family, friends, healthcare providers, and other parents.
- **Focusing on the Positive:**

- o Take time to celebrate the milestones of your pregnancy. Whether it's hearing your baby's heartbeat for the first time, feeling the first kicks, or seeing your baby on an ultrasound, these moments can bring immense joy and help reinforce the positive aspects of your journey.

Chapter 2: The First Trimester

Physical Changes: Early symptoms like morning sickness, fatigue, and breast tenderness.

Morning Sickness

Morning sickness is one of the most well-known and often earliest symptoms of pregnancy. Despite its name, morning sickness can occur at any time of the day. It is characterized by nausea and, in some cases, vomiting. Here are some key aspects of morning sickness:

1. **Timing and Duration:**
   - o Morning sickness typically begins around the sixth week of pregnancy and often subsides by the end of the first trimester. However, some women may experience it earlier, and for others, it can persist longer.
2. **Severity:**
   - o The severity of morning sickness can vary greatly. Some women experience mild nausea, while others may suffer from frequent vomiting that can lead to dehydration and weight loss. In severe cases, a condition known as hyperemesis gravidarum may develop, requiring medical intervention.
3. **Triggers:**
   - o Certain foods, smells, or even the thought of eating can trigger nausea. It can be helpful to identify and avoid your specific triggers to manage symptoms better.
4. **Management:**

- o Eating small, frequent meals instead of three large ones can help keep nausea at bay. Foods that are bland, dry, and easy to digest, such as crackers or toast, are often recommended. Staying hydrated is crucial, so sipping water, ginger tea, or clear broths can be beneficial.
- o Some women find relief through natural remedies like ginger supplements or acupressure bands. However, it's important to consult with a healthcare provider before trying any new treatments.

Fatigue

Fatigue is another common early symptom of pregnancy, often starting as early as the first few weeks after conception. The body undergoes significant changes and increased hormone production, which can contribute to feelings of exhaustion. Key points about fatigue in early pregnancy include:

1. **Hormonal Influence:**
   - o The hormone progesterone rises rapidly in early pregnancy. While essential for maintaining the pregnancy, it also has a sedative effect, which can lead to increased tiredness and the need for more sleep.
2. **Increased Energy Demand:**
   - o Your body is working hard to support the developing embryo, increasing energy demands. This can make you feel more tired than usual.
3. **Rest and Sleep:**
   - o Ensuring you get enough rest is crucial. Listen to your body and take naps if needed. Aim for 7-9 hours of sleep each night, and try to maintain a consistent sleep schedule.
4. **Nutrition and Hydration:**
   - o Eating a balanced diet rich in iron, protein, and other essential nutrients can help combat fatigue.

Staying well-hydrated is also important, as dehydration can exacerbate feelings of tiredness.

5. **Exercise:**
   - Engaging in light to moderate exercise, such as walking or prenatal yoga, can boost your energy levels and improve your overall well-being. However, it's important to avoid overexertion and consult your healthcare provider before starting any new exercise regimen.

Breast Tenderness

Breast tenderness is another early sign of pregnancy, often noticeable within the first few weeks. This symptom occurs due to hormonal changes and increased blood flow to the breast tissue. Key points about breast tenderness include:

1. **Hormonal Changes:**
   - The hormones estrogen and progesterone increase significantly in early pregnancy, preparing the breasts for lactation. This hormonal surge can make the breasts feel sore, sensitive, and swollen.
2. **Changes in Texture:**
   - Your breasts may feel fuller or heavier, and you might notice changes in the texture of the breast tissue. The nipples can also become more sensitive or even painful to the touch.
3. **Appearance:**
   - The areolas (the dark area around the nipples) may darken and enlarge. You might also see more pronounced veins on the surface of your breasts due to increased blood flow.
4. **Support and Comfort:**
   - Wearing a well-fitting, supportive bra can help alleviate discomfort. Many women find that soft, non-underwire bras or maternity bras provide the best support during this time.

- o Using breast pads can help with nipple sensitivity and prevent irritation from clothing.

5. **Warm Compresses:**
   - o Applying warm compresses or taking warm showers can provide relief from breast pain and tenderness. Some women also find cold packs helpful, so it's worth experimenting to see what works best for you.

Coping with Early Symptoms

While these early symptoms of pregnancy can be uncomfortable, there are several strategies to manage and alleviate them:

1. **Healthy Diet:**
   - o Eating a balanced diet with plenty of fruits, vegetables, whole grains, and lean proteins can support your energy levels and overall health. Avoiding caffeine and sugary snacks can also help manage fatigue and nausea.

2. **Hydration:**
   - o Drink plenty of water throughout the day to stay hydrated. Dehydration can worsen symptoms like fatigue and nausea.

3. **Prenatal Vitamins:**
   - o Taking prenatal vitamins as recommended by your healthcare provider ensures you get essential nutrients, such as folic acid, iron, and calcium, which support your body and your baby's development.

4. **Regular Check-ups:**
   - o Regular prenatal visits allow your healthcare provider to monitor your symptoms and provide guidance on managing them effectively. They can also identify and address any complications early on.

5. **Listening to Your Body:**

- o Pay attention to your body's signals and rest when needed. It's important to be gentle with yourself during this time and prioritize your well-being.
6. **Support System:**
   - o Lean on your partner, family, and friends for support. Sharing your experiences and feelings with loved ones can provide emotional comfort and practical assistance.

Health Tips: Nutrition, exercise, and avoiding harmful substances.

Maintaining a healthy lifestyle during pregnancy is crucial for the well-being of both you and your baby. Focusing on proper nutrition, regular exercise, and avoiding harmful substances can help ensure a healthy pregnancy and a strong start for your child. Here are some detailed health tips on these essential aspects.

Nutrition

Good nutrition during pregnancy is vital for your baby's growth and development. Eating a balanced diet ensures that you get the necessary nutrients to support both your health and your baby's. Here are some key points to consider:

1. **Essential Nutrients:**
o **Folic Acid:**
- Folic acid is crucial for preventing neural tube defects. It is recommended to consume at least 400-600 micrograms of folic acid daily, which can be found in leafy greens, citrus fruits, beans, and fortified cereals.
o **Iron:**
- Iron supports the increased blood volume during pregnancy and helps prevent anemia. Good sources of iron include lean meats, poultry, fish, beans, and iron-fortified cereals. Pairing iron-rich foods with vitamin C-rich foods (like oranges or tomatoes) can enhance iron absorption.

- o **Calcium:**
- Calcium is important for the development of your baby's bones and teeth. Aim for 1,000 milligrams of calcium per day from sources such as dairy products, fortified plant milks, tofu, and leafy green vegetables.
- o **Protein:**
- Protein is essential for your baby's growth, especially during the second and third trimesters. Include a variety of protein sources like lean meats, poultry, fish, eggs, beans, and nuts.
- o **Omega-3 Fatty Acids:**
- Omega-3s, particularly DHA, support brain and eye development. Good sources include fatty fish like salmon, flaxseeds, chia seeds, and walnuts.

2. **Balanced Diet:**

- o **Fruits and Vegetables:**
- Aim for at least five servings of fruits and vegetables each day. These provide essential vitamins, minerals, and fiber.
- o **Whole Grains:**
- Choose whole grains over refined grains to ensure you get more fiber and nutrients. Whole grains include brown rice, whole wheat bread, oats, and quinoa.
- o **Healthy Fats:**
- Include healthy fats from sources like avocados, nuts, seeds, and olive oil, which are important for your baby's development.

3. **Hydration:**

- o Drink plenty of water throughout the day to stay hydrated. Proper hydration supports your increased blood volume and helps prevent common pregnancy-related issues like constipation and urinary tract infections.

4. **Prenatal Vitamins:**

- o Taking a prenatal vitamin can help fill any nutritional gaps in your diet. Ensure your prenatal vitamin contains folic acid, iron, calcium, and other essential nutrients. Consult your healthcare provider to choose the right one for you.

Exercise

Regular exercise during pregnancy offers numerous benefits, including improved mood, better sleep, reduced aches and pains, and preparation for labor and delivery. However, it's important to choose safe and appropriate exercises. Here are some tips:

1. **Types of Exercise:**
   - **Walking:**
     - Walking is a safe and easy way to get your daily exercise. Aim for at least 30 minutes of moderate-intensity walking most days of the week.
   - **Swimming:**
     - Swimming and water aerobics are excellent low-impact exercises that can help alleviate joint pain and swelling while providing a full-body workout.
   - **Prenatal Yoga:**
     - Prenatal yoga helps improve flexibility, strength, and relaxation. It also focuses on breathing techniques that can be beneficial during labor.
   - **Strength Training:**
     - Light strength training can help maintain muscle tone and support your changing body. Focus on using light weights and performing exercises with proper form to avoid injury.
2. **Exercise Guidelines:**
   - **Listen to Your Body:**
     - Pay attention to your body's signals and avoid overexertion. If you feel pain, dizziness, or shortness of breath, stop exercising and rest.
   - **Stay Hydrated:**
     - Drink water before, during, and after exercise to stay hydrated.
   - **Avoid High-Risk Activities:**
     - Avoid activities with a high risk of falling or abdominal trauma, such as contact sports, horseback riding, and skiing.

- o **Warm-Up and Cool Down:**
- ▪ Always start with a warm-up to prepare your body for exercise and finish with a cool down to gradually lower your heart rate.

3. **Consult Your Healthcare Provider:**
- o Before starting any new exercise regimen, consult your healthcare provider to ensure it's safe for you and your pregnancy. They can provide personalized recommendations based on your health and pregnancy status.

Avoiding Harmful Substances

Avoiding harmful substances during pregnancy is critical to ensure the health and safety of both you and your baby. Here are some key substances to avoid:

1. **Alcohol:**
- o There is no known safe level of alcohol consumption during pregnancy. Drinking alcohol can lead to fetal alcohol spectrum disorders (FASDs), which can cause developmental delays and birth defects. It's best to abstain from alcohol entirely.
2. **Tobacco:**
- o Smoking or using tobacco products during pregnancy increases the risk of preterm birth, low birth weight, and developmental issues. Secondhand smoke is also harmful, so avoid exposure to smoke-filled environments.
3. **Caffeine:**
- o Limit caffeine intake to 200-300 milligrams per day (about one 12-ounce cup of coffee). Excessive caffeine consumption can increase the risk of miscarriage and preterm birth.
4. **Medications and Supplements:**

o   Consult your healthcare provider before taking any medications, including over-the-counter drugs and supplements. Some medications can be harmful to your developing baby.

5. **Illicit Drugs:**

o   Using illegal drugs during pregnancy can lead to severe complications, including preterm birth, low birth weight, and developmental issues. Seek help from a healthcare provider if you need assistance quitting.

6. **Environmental Toxins:**

o   Avoid exposure to harmful chemicals, such as pesticides, lead, and household cleaners with strong fumes. Opt for natural cleaning products and ensure good ventilation when using chemicals.

7. **Certain Foods:**

o   Some foods pose risks during pregnancy and should be avoided, including:

- **Raw or Undercooked Meat and Fish:**
- These can contain harmful bacteria or parasites. Ensure all meat and fish are thoroughly cooked.
- **Unpasteurized Dairy Products:**
- Unpasteurized milk, cheese, and other dairy products can harbor harmful bacteria like Listeria.
- **Certain Fish High in Mercury:**
- Limit consumption of high-mercury fish like shark, swordfish, king mackerel, and tilefish. Opt for lower-mercury options like salmon, shrimp, and catfish.

Prenatal Care: First prenatal visit, necessary tests, and tracking your pregnancy.

Prenatal care is essential for ensuring a healthy pregnancy and a safe delivery. Regular check-ups, necessary tests, and tracking your pregnancy help monitor your health and your baby's development. Here's an in-depth look at what to expect during your first prenatal visit, the necessary tests throughout your pregnancy, and how to track your pregnancy effectively.

First Prenatal Visit

The first prenatal visit is usually scheduled around 8 to 12 weeks of pregnancy, although it can happen earlier if you have any concerns or health conditions. This visit is crucial for establishing your baseline health and planning your prenatal care. Here's what typically happens during the first prenatal visit:

1. **Medical History Review:**
   o Your healthcare provider will take a detailed medical history, including information about your menstrual cycle, past pregnancies, medical conditions, medications, allergies, and family health history. This helps identify any potential risks or necessary precautions.
2. **Physical Examination:**
   o A thorough physical exam is performed, which may include measuring your weight and height, checking your blood pressure, and assessing your overall health. A pelvic exam and Pap smear might also be conducted to check for any abnormalities.
3. **Blood Tests:**
   o Blood tests are performed to determine your blood type, Rh factor, and to screen for anemia. These tests also check for infectious diseases like HIV, hepatitis B, syphilis, and immunity to rubella and chickenpox.
4. **Urine Tests:**
   o Urine samples are collected to check for infections, protein levels, and glucose levels, which can indicate conditions like urinary tract infections, kidney issues, or gestational diabetes.
5. **Dating Ultrasound:**
   o An early ultrasound may be performed to confirm the pregnancy, determine the due date, and check the baby's heartbeat. This helps ensure the pregnancy is progressing normally.

6. **Health and Lifestyle Discussion:**
o   Your provider will discuss healthy lifestyle choices, including nutrition, exercise, and avoiding harmful substances. They may also address any concerns you have and provide guidance on managing pregnancy symptoms.
7. **Prenatal Vitamins:**
o   You will be advised to take prenatal vitamins, particularly those containing folic acid, iron, and calcium, to support your baby's development and your health.
8. **Schedule Future Visits:**
o   Regular prenatal visits will be scheduled, typically every four weeks during the first and second trimesters, every two weeks during the third trimester until 36 weeks, and then weekly until delivery.

Necessary Tests During Pregnancy

Throughout your pregnancy, several tests are conducted to monitor your health and your baby's development. These tests help detect any potential issues early and ensure timely intervention if necessary. Here are some common tests you can expect:

1. **Blood Pressure and Urine Tests:**
o   At each prenatal visit, your blood pressure and urine will be checked to monitor for conditions like preeclampsia and gestational diabetes.
2. **Genetic Screening Tests:**
o   These tests assess the risk of certain genetic conditions. They may include:
- **First Trimester Screening:**
- A combination of a blood test and ultrasound (nuchal translucency) performed between 11 and 14 weeks to assess the risk of chromosomal abnormalities like Down syndrome.
- **Non-Invasive Prenatal Testing (NIPT):**
- A blood test performed as early as 10 weeks to screen for chromosomal disorders.

- **Second Trimester Screening (Quad Screen):**
- A blood test performed between 15 and 22 weeks to measure levels of specific substances in your blood and assess the risk of neural tube defects and chromosomal abnormalities.

3. **Anatomy Ultrasound:**
   - Typically performed between 18 and 22 weeks, this detailed ultrasound examines the baby's anatomy to ensure everything is developing normally. It can also reveal the baby's sex if you wish to know.

4. **Glucose Screening Test:**
   - Conducted between 24 and 28 weeks to screen for gestational diabetes. You will drink a sugary solution, and your blood sugar levels will be tested an hour later.

5. **Group B Streptococcus (GBS) Test:**
   - Performed between 35 and 37 weeks to check for GBS bacteria in the vagina and rectum. If positive, you will receive antibiotics during labor to prevent transmission to the baby.

6. **Additional Tests:**
   - Depending on your health and pregnancy, additional tests such as amniocentesis, chorionic villus sampling (CVS), or fetal echocardiography might be recommended.

Tracking Your Pregnancy

Tracking your pregnancy helps you stay informed about your baby's development and your health. Here are some ways to effectively track your pregnancy:

1. **Pregnancy Apps:**
   - There are numerous pregnancy apps available that provide weekly updates on your baby's development, track your symptoms, and remind you of upcoming appointments. Examples include What to Expect, The Bump, and BabyCenter.

2. **Pregnancy Journal:**
   - Keeping a pregnancy journal allows you to document your experiences, emotions, and milestones. This can be a great keepsake and help you reflect on your journey.
3. **Prenatal Visit Schedule:**
   - Keep a calendar or use an app to track your prenatal visit schedule and any recommended tests. This ensures you don't miss any important appointments.
4. **Symptom Tracking:**
   - Note any symptoms or changes you experience, such as morning sickness, fatigue, or swelling. This information can be helpful for your healthcare provider to monitor your pregnancy and address any concerns.
5. **Weight and Nutrition Log:**
   - Track your weight gain and nutritional intake to ensure you are meeting your dietary needs. This can help prevent excessive weight gain and ensure you are getting the necessary nutrients for your baby's growth.
6. **Exercise Routine:**
   - Keep a log of your exercise routine to stay motivated and ensure you are getting regular physical activity. This can include walking, prenatal yoga, or any other recommended exercises.
7. **Baby Movements:**
   - As your pregnancy progresses, tracking your baby's movements can provide reassurance of their well-being. Count kicks and note any significant changes in activity levels.

Chapter 3: Exercise During Pregnancy

Benefits of Exercise: Why staying active is important.

1. Improved Physical Health

A. Cardiovascular Health:

- **Enhanced Circulation:**
  o Regular exercise improves blood flow, reducing the risk of developing varicose veins and swelling in the legs and feet.
- **Heart Health:**
  o Staying active strengthens the heart, reducing the risk of pregnancy-induced hypertension (high blood pressure) and preeclampsia.

B. Weight Management:

- **Healthy Weight Gain:**
  o Exercise helps regulate weight gain during pregnancy, ensuring it stays within a healthy range. This can prevent complications such as gestational diabetes and large-for-gestational-age babies.

C. Reduced Risk of Gestational Diabetes:

- **Blood Sugar Control:**
  o Regular physical activity helps regulate blood sugar levels, reducing the risk of developing gestational diabetes, a common pregnancy complication.

D. Eased Digestive Issues:

- **Relief from Constipation:**
  o Exercise stimulates intestinal function, helping to prevent and alleviate constipation, a common issue during pregnancy.

2. Enhanced Mental Health

A. Reduced Stress and Anxiety:

- **Mood Boost:**
  - Exercise stimulates the release of endorphins, natural mood elevators that can help reduce stress, anxiety, and depression.
- **Improved Sleep:**
  - Physical activity can improve sleep quality, helping pregnant women get the rest they need despite the discomforts of pregnancy.

B. Increased Energy Levels:

- **Combat Fatigue:**
  - Regular exercise boosts energy levels, helping to combat the fatigue that often accompanies pregnancy.

3. Easier Pregnancy and Labor

A. Alleviation of Common Pregnancy Discomforts:

- **Reduced Back Pain:**
  - Strengthening the muscles, especially the core and back, can help alleviate the back pain that often accompanies pregnancy.
- **Improved Posture:**
  - Exercise helps improve posture, reducing strain on the lower back.

B. Preparation for Labor:

- **Strength and Stamina:**

- o Regular physical activity enhances overall strength and stamina, which can be incredibly beneficial during labor and delivery.
- **Flexibility and Endurance:**
- o Exercises like prenatal yoga improve flexibility and endurance, making it easier to cope with labor and reducing the likelihood of complications.

C. Faster Recovery Postpartum:

- **Quicker Postpartum Recovery:**
- o Women who exercise during pregnancy often experience a quicker recovery postpartum, with a faster return to pre-pregnancy fitness levels.

4. Healthy Baby Development

A. Optimal Birth Weight:

- **Healthy Weight Gain:**
- o Maintaining an active lifestyle contributes to a healthy weight gain for the baby, reducing the risk of complications during delivery.
- **Reduced Risk of Macrosomia:**
- o Exercise helps prevent excessive fetal weight gain, reducing the risk of macrosomia (having a very large baby), which can complicate delivery.

B. Enhanced Brain Development:

- **Increased Blood Flow:**
  - o Regular exercise improves blood flow to the placenta, providing the baby with more oxygen and nutrients, which can enhance brain development.

5. Social Benefits

A. Support and Community:

- **Group Activities:**
    - Participating in prenatal exercise classes provides a sense of community and support from other pregnant women.
- **Shared Experiences:**
    - Engaging in group activities allows for the sharing of experiences, tips, and encouragement, fostering a supportive environment.

B. Improved Relationship with Partner:

- **Bonding Time:**
    - Exercise can provide a bonding opportunity for couples, especially if they participate in activities together, such as walking or prenatal yoga.
- **Shared Health Goals:**
    - Working out together can strengthen the relationship by fostering shared health goals and mutual support.

6. Types of Safe Exercises

A. Walking:

- **Low-Impact Cardio:**
    - Walking is a safe, low-impact exercise that can be easily incorporated into daily routines. It provides cardiovascular benefits without straining the joints.

B. Swimming:

- **Full-Body Workout:**

- o Swimming offers a full-body workout that is easy on the joints and helps alleviate swelling. The buoyancy of water provides relief from the extra weight of pregnancy.

C. Prenatal Yoga:

- **Flexibility and Relaxation:**
  - o Prenatal yoga improves flexibility, strength, and relaxation. It also teaches breathing techniques that can be beneficial during labor.

D. Strength Training:

- **Muscle Tone:**
  - o Light strength training helps maintain muscle tone and supports the changing body. Focus on using light weights and proper form to avoid injury.

E. Pelvic Floor Exercises:

- **Kegel Exercises:**
  - o Strengthening the pelvic floor muscles can prevent issues like incontinence and support the uterus, bladder, and bowels during and after pregnancy.

Safe Exercises: Recommended workouts for each trimester.

First Trimester (Weeks 1-12)

During the first trimester, it's important to establish a consistent exercise routine while being mindful of your changing body and energy levels. Focus on low-impact exercises that build strength, flexibility, and endurance.

A. Walking:

- **Benefits:**

o   Walking is a low-impact cardiovascular exercise that is easy to incorporate into daily routines. It helps maintain fitness without putting excessive strain on the body.

- **Routine:**

o   Aim for 30 minutes of walking most days of the week. Start with a moderate pace and gradually increase the intensity as you feel comfortable.

B. Swimming:

- **Benefits:**

o   Swimming provides a full-body workout and relieves pressure on the joints. The buoyancy of water supports your growing belly and reduces swelling.

- **Routine:**

o   Swim for 30-45 minutes, three to four times a week. Alternate between different strokes to engage various muscle groups.

C. Prenatal Yoga:

- **Benefits:**

o   Prenatal yoga improves flexibility, strength, and relaxation. It also teaches breathing techniques that can be helpful during labor.

- **Routine:**

o   Attend a prenatal yoga class once or twice a week. Focus on gentle poses that enhance flexibility and reduce stress.

D. Strength Training:

- **Benefits:**

o   Light strength training helps maintain muscle tone and supports your changing body. It also helps prepare for the physical demands of labor and motherhood.

- **Routine:**

- o Use light weights or resistance bands. Perform exercises like bicep curls, tricep extensions, and leg lifts. Aim for two to three sessions per week.

E. Pelvic Floor Exercises:

- **Benefits:**
- o Strengthening the pelvic floor muscles helps prevent issues like incontinence and supports the uterus, bladder, and bowels.
- **Routine:**
- o Perform Kegel exercises daily. Squeeze and hold the pelvic floor muscles for 5-10 seconds, then relax. Repeat 10-15 times.

Second Trimester (Weeks 13-27)

The second trimester is often considered the most comfortable phase of pregnancy. Energy levels typically increase, and morning sickness often subsides. Continue with low-impact exercises and start incorporating more strength and flexibility workouts.

A. Walking:

- **Routine:**
- o Continue with 30-minute walks most days of the week. You can add light hills or stairs to increase the intensity if you feel comfortable.

B. Swimming:

- **Routine:**
- o Maintain swimming sessions of 30-45 minutes, three to four times a week. Focus on maintaining good form and breathing techniques.

C. Prenatal Yoga:

- **Routine:**
  - Attend prenatal yoga classes once or twice a week. Incorporate poses that open the hips, stretch the back, and strengthen the legs.

D. Strength Training:

- **Routine:**
  - Use light to moderate weights or resistance bands. Include exercises like squats, lunges, and seated rows. Perform two to three sessions per week, with 10-12 repetitions per set.

E. Pelvic Floor Exercises:

- **Routine:**
  - Continue daily Kegel exercises. Incorporate variations such as quick squeezes and longer holds to strengthen different muscle fibers.

F. Pilates:

- **Benefits:**
  - Prenatal Pilates focuses on core strength, balance, and flexibility, helping to support the growing belly and reduce back pain.
- **Routine:**
  - Attend a prenatal Pilates class once a week or follow a guided routine at home.

Third Trimester (Weeks 28-40)

In the third trimester, focus on maintaining your fitness level while preparing for labor and delivery. Choose exercises that promote relaxation, reduce discomfort, and support your changing body.

A. Walking:

- **Routine:**
  - o Continue with 20-30 minute walks most days of the week. Opt for flat, even surfaces to avoid falls and maintain a moderate pace.

B. Swimming:

- **Routine:**
  - o Maintain swimming sessions of 30 minutes, two to three times a week. Swimming is particularly beneficial in the third trimester as it alleviates pressure on the joints and reduces swelling.

C. Prenatal Yoga:

- **Routine:**
  - o Attend prenatal yoga classes once a week. Focus on gentle stretches, relaxation techniques, and breathing exercises that can be useful during labor.

D. Strength Training:

- **Routine:**
  - o Use light weights or bodyweight exercises. Include modified squats, wall push-ups, and seated resistance band exercises. Perform two sessions per week with 8-10 repetitions per set.

E. Pelvic Floor Exercises:

- **Routine:**
  - o Continue daily Kegel exercises. Practice different variations to maintain pelvic floor strength and flexibility.

F. Gentle Stretching:

- **Benefits:**

- o Stretching helps relieve muscle tension, improve flexibility, and reduce pregnancy-related discomforts such as back pain and sciatica.
- **Routine:**
  - o Incorporate gentle stretching routines daily. Focus on stretches for the back, hips, and legs.

G. Birthing Ball Exercises:

- **Benefits:**
  - o Using a birthing ball can help open the pelvis, improve posture, and relieve lower back pain. It can also be used for labor preparation exercises.
- **Routine:**
  - o Sit on the birthing ball and practice gentle bouncing, hip circles, and pelvic tilts for 10-15 minutes a day.

Safety Tips for Exercising During Pregnancy

- **Consult Your Healthcare Provider:**
  - o Always consult with your healthcare provider before starting or continuing any exercise regimen during pregnancy.
- **Listen to Your Body:**
  - o Pay attention to your body's signals. If you feel pain, dizziness, shortness of breath, or excessive fatigue, stop exercising and rest.
- **Stay Hydrated:**
  - o Drink plenty of water before, during, and after exercise to stay hydrated.
- **Avoid Overheating:**
  - o Wear breathable, loose-fitting clothing and exercise in a cool, well-ventilated environment to avoid overheating.
- **Use Proper Technique:**

- o Focus on maintaining proper form and technique to prevent injuries. Consider working with a prenatal fitness instructor if you're unsure about certain exercises.

Exercise Precautions: Activities to avoid and when to consult your doctor.

Activities to Avoid

A. High-Impact and Contact Sports:

- **Examples:**
- o Basketball, soccer, hockey, and other sports that involve physical contact or a high risk of falling.
- **Risks:**
- o These activities can lead to abdominal trauma, falls, and injuries, which could harm both you and your baby.

B. Activities with a High Risk of Falling:

- **Examples:**
- o Skiing, snowboarding, horseback riding, gymnastics, and cycling (particularly in later stages of pregnancy).
- **Risks:**
- o The risk of falls increases as your center of gravity shifts with your growing belly, making these activities unsafe.

C. Scuba Diving:

- **Risks:**
- o Scuba diving is dangerous during pregnancy due to the risk of decompression sickness and gas embolism, which can affect the baby.

D. Hot Yoga and Hot Pilates:

- **Risks:**
  - These activities involve high temperatures, which can lead to overheating and dehydration, posing risks to both mother and baby.

E. Heavy Weightlifting:

- **Risks:**
  - Lifting heavy weights can strain your joints and pelvic floor. It's safer to use lighter weights with more repetitions or to focus on bodyweight exercises.

F. Exercises Lying Flat on Your Back After the First Trimester:

- **Risks:**
- Lying flat on your back can compress the vena cava, a major vein that returns blood to the heart, potentially reducing blood flow to the baby and causing dizziness.

G. High-Intensity Interval Training (HIIT):

- **Risks:**
  - High-intensity exercises can lead to overexertion, dehydration, and overheating. Opt for moderate-intensity workouts instead.

H. Deep Squats and Lunges:

- **Risks:**
  - Deep squats and lunges can increase pelvic pressure and potentially lead to pelvic instability, especially if you have a history of pelvic pain.

When to Consult Your Doctor

A. Pre-existing Medical Conditions:

- **Conditions:**
  - If you have any pre-existing medical conditions such as heart disease, asthma, hypertension, or diabetes, consult your doctor before starting or continuing an exercise regimen.

B. Pregnancy Complications:

- **Conditions:**
  - If you have pregnancy-related complications such as preeclampsia, placenta previa, cervical insufficiency, or a history of preterm labor, seek medical advice regarding safe exercise options.

C. Unusual Symptoms During Exercise:

- **Symptoms:**
  - Vaginal bleeding or spotting
  - Severe abdominal pain or cramping
  - Sudden swelling in the face, hands, or feet
  - Dizziness, fainting, or shortness of breath
  - Severe headaches
  - Chest pain
  - Muscle weakness affecting balance
  - Decreased fetal movement
- **Action:**
  - Stop exercising immediately and contact your healthcare provider if you experience any of these symptoms during or after exercise.

D. Changes in Pregnancy Status:

- **Situations:**
  - If you experience significant changes in your pregnancy status, such as bed rest recommendations, significant weight gain or loss, or changes in fetal development, discuss with your doctor how to adjust your exercise routine accordingly.

E. Post-Surgical Concerns:

- **Situations:**
  - If you've had recent surgery, such as a cesarean section or any other abdominal surgery, consult your healthcare provider about appropriate post-surgery exercise routines and timelines.

General Safety Tips for Exercising During Pregnancy

A. Warm Up and Cool Down:

- **Importance:**
  - Always start with a gentle warm-up to prepare your body for exercise and end with a cool-down to gradually lower your heart rate and stretch your muscles.

B. Stay Hydrated:

- **Tip:**
  - Drink plenty of water before, during, and after exercise to stay hydrated and prevent overheating.

C. Wear Comfortable Clothing:

- **Tip:**

o Wear breathable, loose-fitting clothing and a supportive sports bra to accommodate your changing body and provide necessary support.

D. Avoid Overheating:

- **Tip:**
  - o Exercise in a cool, well-ventilated environment, and avoid activities that can lead to overheating, especially in hot and humid conditions.

E. Monitor Your Intensity:

- **Guideline:**
  - o Use the "talk test" to gauge intensity—if you can hold a conversation comfortably while exercising, the intensity is appropriate. Avoid pushing yourself to the point of breathlessness.

F. Listen to Your Body:

- **Guideline:**
  - o Pay attention to your body's signals and stop exercising if you feel pain, discomfort, or fatigue. Rest is equally important during pregnancy.

G. Modify Exercises as Needed:

- **Tip:**
  - o As your pregnancy progresses, modify exercises to accommodate your growing belly and changing body. Focus on maintaining proper form and avoiding exercises that cause discomfort.

H. Use Proper Footwear:

- **Tip:**

      o   Wear supportive shoes that provide good stability and cushioning to reduce the risk of injury and support your joints.

Chapter 4: Pregnancy Nutrition

Essential Nutrients: Key vitamins and minerals for a healthy pregnancy.

1. Folic Acid (Folate)

Importance:

- Folic acid is crucial for neural tube development, which forms the baby's brain and spinal cord in the early weeks of pregnancy.
- Adequate folate intake reduces the risk of neural tube defects such as spina bifida and anencephaly.

Food Sources:

- Leafy green vegetables (spinach, kale)
- Legumes (beans, lentils)
- Citrus fruits (oranges, grapefruits)
- Fortified grains (bread, cereal)

Recommended Intake:

- 600 micrograms (mcg) per day for pregnant women
- Some women may require higher doses, so consult with your healthcare provider.

2. Iron

Importance:

- Iron is essential for the production of hemoglobin, which carries oxygen to your tissues and to your baby.
- During pregnancy, blood volume increases, and iron helps prevent anemia and supports the baby's growth and development.

Food Sources:

- Lean red meat (beef, pork)
- Poultry (chicken, turkey)
- Fish (especially shellfish)
- Beans and lentils
- Fortified cereals
- Dark, leafy greens (spinach, kale)

Recommended Intake:

- 27 milligrams (mg) per day for pregnant women
- Iron supplements may be recommended if dietary intake is insufficient or if you develop anemia.

3. Calcium

Importance:

- Calcium is essential for the development of your baby's bones, teeth, muscles, and nerves.
- It also helps maintain your own bone health and prevents bone density loss during pregnancy and breastfeeding.

Food Sources:

- Dairy products (milk, yogurt, cheese)
- Fortified plant-based milks (soy, almond)
- Leafy green vegetables (collard greens, bok choy)
- Tofu

- Canned fish with bones (sardines, salmon)

Recommended Intake:

- 1000 mg per day for pregnant women aged 19-50 years
- Some women may require additional calcium supplements, especially if dietary intake is inadequate.

4. Vitamin D

Importance:

- Vitamin D helps the body absorb calcium, supporting bone health and development.
- It also plays a role in immune function and may reduce the risk of certain pregnancy complications.

Food Sources:

- Fatty fish (salmon, mackerel, tuna)
- Fortified dairy products (milk, yogurt)
- Fortified cereals
- Egg yolks
- Sunlight exposure stimulates vitamin D production in the skin.

Recommended Intake:

- 600 International Units (IU) per day for pregnant women
- Some women may require higher doses if they have limited sun exposure or vitamin D deficiency.

5. Omega-3 Fatty Acids

Importance:

- Omega-3 fatty acids, particularly DHA (docosahexaenoic acid), are crucial for the development of the baby's brain and eyes.
- They also support maternal heart health and may reduce the risk of preterm birth and postpartum depression.

Food Sources:

- Fatty fish (salmon, trout, sardines)
- Fish oil supplements (choose ones labeled as safe for pregnancy)
- Flaxseeds and chia seeds
- Walnuts

Recommended Intake:

- Aim for at least 200-300 mg of DHA per day during pregnancy.
- Consider taking a fish oil supplement if dietary intake is insufficient, but consult with your healthcare provider first.

6. Iodine

Importance:

- Iodine is essential for thyroid function, which regulates metabolism and supports fetal brain development.
- Severe iodine deficiency during pregnancy can lead to intellectual disabilities and growth retardation in the baby.

Food Sources:

- Iodized salt
- Seafood (cod, shrimp, seaweed)
- Dairy products (milk, yogurt, cheese)
- Eggs

Recommended Intake:

- 220 micrograms (mcg) per day for pregnant women
- Most prenatal vitamins contain iodine, but check the label to ensure adequate intake.

7. Vitamin C

Importance:

- Vitamin C is important for collagen formation, which supports the development of the baby's bones, cartilage, and connective tissues.
- It also boosts the immune system and enhances iron absorption.

Food Sources:

- Citrus fruits (oranges, grapefruits)
- Berries (strawberries, blueberries)
- Kiwi
- Bell peppers
- Tomatoes

Recommended Intake:

- 85 mg per day for pregnant women
- Aim to include a variety of vitamin C-rich foods in your diet to meet daily needs.

8. Vitamin B12

Importance:

- Vitamin B12 is essential for nervous system function and the formation of red blood cells.
- Adequate intake is important for the baby's brain and nervous system development.

Food Sources:

- Animal products (meat, fish, poultry, eggs, dairy)
- Fortified plant-based foods (nutritional yeast, fortified cereals, plant-based milk)

Recommended Intake:

- 2.6 micrograms (mcg) per day for pregnant women
- If following a vegetarian or vegan diet, consider taking a B12 supplement or eating fortified foods to ensure adequate intake.

Cravings and Aversions: Managing cravings and dealing with food aversions.

Managing Cravings:

1. Understand the Cause:

- Recognize that cravings are a normal part of pregnancy, often influenced by hormonal changes and nutrient needs. Cravings may also be triggered by emotions, cultural influences, or memories.

2. Practice Moderation:

- It's okay to indulge in your cravings occasionally, but aim for moderation to maintain a balanced diet. Choose healthier options when possible, such as dark chocolate instead of sugary treats or fruit instead of candy.

3. Satisfy Nutrient Needs:

- Cravings can sometimes indicate a need for specific nutrients. Pay attention to the type of foods you crave and try to incorporate nutrient-rich alternatives. For example, craving red meat may signal a need for iron.

4. Plan Ahead:

- Keep healthier alternatives on hand to satisfy cravings without compromising nutrition. Stock up on nutritious snacks like nuts, fruits, yogurt, or whole-grain crackers to curb cravings.

5. Stay Hydrated:

- Sometimes thirst can be mistaken for hunger or cravings. Drink plenty of water throughout the day to stay hydrated, which may help reduce cravings.

6. Distract Yourself:

- Engage in activities that distract you from cravings, such as going for a walk, practicing relaxation techniques, or pursuing a hobby. Sometimes cravings diminish when you focus your attention elsewhere.

Dealing with Food Aversions:

1. Identify Triggers:

- Pay attention to specific smells, tastes, or textures that trigger aversions. Understanding your triggers can help you avoid them or find alternatives.

2. Experiment with Preparation Methods:

- Try preparing foods in different ways to see if it changes their taste or texture. For example, if you're averse to certain vegetables raw, try cooking or steaming them.

3. Focus on Nutrient-Rich Foods:

- If you're experiencing aversions to certain foods, focus on consuming nutrient-rich alternatives that provide similar benefits. For example, if you can't tolerate dairy, opt for calcium-fortified plant-based milk.

4. Listen to Your Body:

- Respect your body's cues and eat what feels tolerable and nourishing. Don't force yourself to eat foods that make you feel nauseous or uncomfortable.

5. Be Flexible with Meal Planning:

- Accept that your tastes may change throughout pregnancy and be flexible with meal planning. Embrace variety and experiment with new foods to find what works for you.

6. Seek Support:

- Communicate your food aversions to your partner, family, or friends, so they can offer support and understanding. Sharing your experiences can help alleviate stress and anxiety related to food aversions.

7. Consider Prenatal Supplements:

- If you're unable to tolerate certain foods due to aversions, consider taking prenatal supplements to ensure you're getting essential nutrients. Consult with your healthcare provider to determine the appropriate supplements for your needs.

Chapter 5: Emotional Well-being

Mental Health: Managing stress, anxiety, and mood swings.

1. Practice Relaxation Techniques:

A. Deep Breathing:

- Take slow, deep breaths to calm your mind and body. Practice deep breathing exercises regularly, especially when feeling anxious or stressed.

B. Progressive Muscle Relaxation:

- Tense and then relax each muscle group in your body, starting from your toes and working your way up to your head. This technique can help release tension and promote relaxation.

C. Mindfulness Meditation:

- Engage in mindfulness meditation to focus your attention on the present moment and cultivate a

> sense of calm and acceptance. Mindfulness
> practices can reduce stress and anxiety levels.

2. Stay Active:

A. Gentle Exercise:

- Engage in gentle exercises such as walking, prenatal yoga, or swimming. Physical activity releases endorphins, which can improve mood and reduce stress.

B. Practice Prenatal Yoga:

- Prenatal yoga combines gentle stretches, breathing exercises, and meditation to promote relaxation and reduce stress. It also helps prepare the body for labor and delivery.

3. Prioritize Self-Care:

A. Get Adequate Rest:

- Prioritize sleep and rest, especially during the first and third trimesters when fatigue may be more pronounced. Aim for 7-9 hours of quality sleep per night.

B. Establish a Routine:

- Establish a daily routine that includes time for relaxation, hobbies, and activities you enjoy. Having a structured schedule can provide a sense of stability and control.

C. Take Breaks:

- Listen to your body and take breaks when needed. Avoid overexertion and give yourself permission to rest and recharge.

4. Seek Support:

A. Talk to Your Partner:

- Communicate openly with your partner about your feelings, concerns, and needs. Lean on each other for support and understanding during this time of change.

B. Connect with Other Expectant Mothers:

- Join a prenatal support group or attend childbirth education classes to connect with other expectant mothers. Sharing experiences and concerns with others who are going through similar experiences can provide validation and support.

C. Consider Therapy:

- If you're struggling to cope with stress, anxiety, or mood swings, consider seeking professional help from a therapist or counselor who specializes in perinatal mental health. Therapy can provide valuable coping strategies and emotional support.

5. Practice Healthy Coping Strategies:

A. Express Yourself:

- Journaling, writing, or creating art can be therapeutic ways to express your emotions and process your thoughts.

B. Limit Stressors:

- Identify sources of stress in your life and take steps to minimize or eliminate them whenever possible. Delegate tasks, set boundaries, and prioritize self-care.

C. Focus on Positive Self-Talk:

- Challenge negative thoughts and replace them with positive affirmations. Practice self-compassion and acknowledge your strengths and accomplishments.

6. Communicate with Your Healthcare Provider:

A. Be Honest About Your Feelings:

- Don't hesitate to discuss your mental health concerns with your healthcare provider. They can offer guidance, support, and resources to help you cope.

B. Explore Treatment Options:

- If necessary, explore treatment options such as therapy or medication under the guidance of your healthcare provider. It's essential to prioritize your mental health during pregnancy.

Support Systems: The importance of a support network.

1. Emotional Support:

A. Validation and Understanding:

- A supportive network of family, friends, and partners can provide validation and understanding during times of emotional upheaval. They can empathize with your experiences and offer reassurance and comfort.

B. Coping with Stress and Anxiety:

- Pregnancy can be a time of heightened emotions, stress, and anxiety. Having someone to talk to and lean on can help alleviate feelings of isolation and overwhelm.

C. Processing Complex Emotions:

- Pregnancy often brings up a range of complex emotions, including excitement, fear, and uncertainty. A supportive network can provide a safe space to express and process these emotions without judgment.

2. Practical Support:

A. Assistance with Daily Tasks:

- As pregnancy progresses, physical discomfort and fatigue may make it challenging to perform daily tasks. A support network can offer practical assistance with household chores, errands, and childcare responsibilities.

B. Accompanying to Appointments:

- Attending prenatal appointments and ultrasounds can be reassuring, but it's not always possible for partners or family members to accompany expectant mothers. Having someone there for support can make these experiences more meaningful and less daunting.

C. Help with Preparations:

- From setting up the nursery to shopping for baby essentials, preparing for the arrival of a new baby can be overwhelming. A support network can lend a helping hand with preparations, easing the burden on expectant mothers.

3. Social Support:

A. Connection and Camaraderie:

- Pregnancy can sometimes feel isolating, especially if you're the first among your friends or family to experience it. Building connections with other expectant mothers through support groups or online forums can provide a sense of camaraderie and shared experiences.

B. Sharing Knowledge and Resources:

- Your support network can offer valuable advice, tips, and resources based on their own experiences with pregnancy and parenting. Whether it's recommendations for healthcare providers, baby gear, or parenting books, their insights can be invaluable.

C. Celebrating Milestones:

- Pregnancy is filled with exciting milestones, from feeling the baby's first kicks to seeing ultrasound images. Sharing these moments with your support network can make them even more memorable and special.

4. Partner Support:

A. Emotional Connection:

- Partners play a crucial role in providing emotional support during pregnancy. They can listen, offer encouragement, and be a source of strength during challenging times.

B. Involvement in Pregnancy:

- Partners can actively participate in pregnancy by attending appointments, helping with household tasks, and offering physical affection and comfort.

C. Strengthening the Relationship:

- Pregnancy is a time of transition for both partners, and navigating this journey together can strengthen the bond between them. Open communication, mutual support, and shared experiences can deepen the connection and lay the foundation for a strong partnership as parents.

Mindfulness and Relaxation: Techniques like meditation and yoga for relaxation.

1. Mindfulness Meditation:

A. Body Scan Meditation:

- Find a comfortable position, either sitting or lying down. Close your eyes and bring your attention to different parts of your body, starting from your toes and gradually moving up to your head. Notice any sensations, tension, or areas of relaxation. Take deep breaths and allow any tension to release with each exhale.

B. Breathing Meditation:

- Sit comfortably with your spine straight and shoulders relaxed. Close your eyes and focus on your breath. Inhale deeply through your nose, feeling your belly expand, and exhale slowly through your mouth, feeling your body relax. Repeat this process, allowing your breath to anchor you in the present moment and calm your mind.

C. Loving-Kindness Meditation:

- Sit quietly and bring to mind someone you love, such as your baby, partner, or a supportive friend. Silently repeat phrases such as "May you be happy, may you be healthy, may you be safe, may you live with ease." Extend these wishes to yourself and then to all beings, cultivating feelings of love, compassion, and connection.

2. Prenatal Yoga:

A. Gentle Stretching:

- Practice gentle stretches that target areas of tension or discomfort, such as the hips, lower back, and shoulders. Focus on slow, mindful movements and deep breathing to release tension and promote relaxation.

B. Modified Poses:

- Choose yoga poses that are safe and comfortable for pregnancy, avoiding deep twists, backbends, and poses that compress the abdomen. Modify poses as needed by using props such as bolsters, blocks, or blankets for support.

C. Pelvic Floor Exercises:

- Incorporate pelvic floor exercises, such as Kegels, into your yoga practice to strengthen the pelvic muscles and prepare for childbirth. Focus on engaging and relaxing the pelvic floor with each breath.

3. Guided Imagery:

A. Visualization:

- Close your eyes and visualize a peaceful and serene place, such as a tranquil beach or a lush forest. Engage all your senses in the imagery, imagining the sights, sounds, smells, and sensations of being in that place. Allow yourself to fully immerse in the experience and let go of any stress or tension.

B. Positive Affirmations:

- Repeat positive affirmations or mantras that resonate with you, such as "I am calm, confident, and capable," or "My body knows how to nurture and support my baby." Use these affirmations to cultivate feelings of empowerment, confidence, and relaxation.

4. Progressive Muscle Relaxation:

A. Body Awareness:

- Start by tensing and then slowly relaxing each muscle group in your body, starting from your toes and moving up to your head. Focus on the sensations of tension and relaxation in each muscle, allowing them to release any built-up tension.

B. Deep Breathing:

- Coordinate your muscle relaxation with deep breathing, inhaling as you tense the muscles and exhaling as you release them. Visualize any stress or tension leaving your body with each exhale, leaving you feeling calm and relaxed.

Routine Check-ups: What to expect at each prenatal visit.

1. First Prenatal Visit (6-8 Weeks):

A. Medical History:

- Your healthcare provider will review your medical history, including any pre-existing conditions, past pregnancies, and family medical history.

B. Physical Examination:

- A physical examination may include measuring your height, weight, blood pressure, and calculating your body mass index (BMI). Your provider may also perform a pelvic exam to assess your reproductive health.

C. Laboratory Tests:

- Blood and urine tests may be ordered to confirm the pregnancy, check for any underlying health conditions, and screen for infections, genetic disorders, and other potential risks.

D. Prenatal Screening:

- You may discuss options for prenatal screening tests, such as ultrasound and blood tests, to assess the risk of chromosomal abnormalities and birth defects.

E. Prenatal Education:

- Your provider will offer information and resources on nutrition, exercise, prenatal vitamins, lifestyle habits, and what to expect during pregnancy.

2. Regular Prenatal Visits (Every 4 Weeks Until 28 Weeks, Then Every 2 Weeks Until 36 Weeks, and Weekly Until Delivery):

A. Physical Assessment:

- At each visit, your healthcare provider will measure your weight, blood pressure, and fundal height (the distance from the pubic bone to the top of the uterus) to monitor the baby's growth and development.

B. Fetal Monitoring:

- Your provider may use a Doppler ultrasound or fetal heart rate monitor to listen to the baby's heartbeat and assess fetal movements and positioning.

C. Screening Tests:

- Depending on your stage of pregnancy, you may undergo additional prenatal screening tests, such as glucose tolerance tests for gestational diabetes, Group B streptococcus (GBS) screening, and fetal anatomy ultrasounds.

D. Addressing Concerns:

- Use this time to discuss any concerns, symptoms, or questions you may have about your pregnancy, labor and delivery, breastfeeding, or postpartum care.

E. Prenatal Education:

- Your provider will continue to offer guidance and education on topics such as nutrition, exercise, childbirth preparation, breastfeeding, newborn care, and postpartum recovery.

3. Third Trimester Visits (Starting at 28 Weeks):

A. Gestational Diabetes Screening:

- Between 24 and 28 weeks, you'll undergo screening for gestational diabetes, which involves drinking a sugary solution and undergoing blood tests to assess your body's ability to process glucose.

B. Group B Streptococcus (GBS) Screening:

- Around 36 weeks, you'll be screened for Group B streptococcus (GBS), a type of bacteria that can be passed to the baby during childbirth and may require antibiotic treatment during labor.

C. Birth Plan Discussion:

- Discuss your birth preferences, including labor and delivery options, pain management strategies, and any special considerations or concerns you may have.

D. Preparation for Labor and Delivery:

- Your provider will discuss signs and symptoms of labor, when to call or go to the hospital, and what to expect during the final weeks of pregnancy.

E. Postpartum Planning:

- Start planning for the postpartum period, including postpartum care, support resources, and newborn care basics.

4. Weekly Visits in Late Pregnancy (Starting at 36 Weeks):

A. Fetal Assessment:

- Your provider will closely monitor fetal growth and well-being, including assessing fetal movement, heart rate, and positioning.

B. Cervical Exam:

- Your provider may perform cervical exams to check for signs of cervical dilation and effacement, which can indicate the onset of labor.

C. Final Preparation:

- Finalize preparations for labor and delivery, including packing your hospital bag, reviewing your birth plan, and confirming arrangements for childcare and support during labor.

D. Emotional Support:

- Use these visits as an opportunity to express any fears, anxieties, or emotional concerns you may have about childbirth and parenthood.

Monitoring Baby's Health: Keeping track of fetal movements and growth.

1. Fetal Movements:

A. Kick Counts:

- Starting around the 28th week of pregnancy, spend some time each day counting your baby's movements. Lie on your left side and pay attention to how long it takes to feel ten distinct movements, such as kicks, rolls, or jabs. Note the time it takes to reach ten movements and report any significant changes to your healthcare provider.

B. Daily Routine:

- Choose a consistent time of day when your baby is typically active, such as after a meal or in the evening, to perform kick counts. Sit or lie quietly and focus on feeling your baby's movements without distractions.

C. Movement Patterns:

- Get to know your baby's typical movement patterns and frequency. While every baby is different, most babies have active periods and periods of rest throughout the day. If you notice a significant decrease in fetal movements or a change in movement patterns, contact your healthcare provider immediately.

2. Fundal Height Measurement:

A. Growth Assessment:

- At each prenatal visit, your healthcare provider will measure your fundal height, which is the distance from the pubic bone to the top of the uterus. Fundal height measurements help assess your baby's growth and development.

B. Growth Chart:

- Your provider will plot your fundal height measurements on a growth chart to track your baby's growth over time. Consistent growth along the expected curve is a positive sign of healthy development.

C. Ultrasound Imaging:

- If there are concerns about fetal growth or development, your provider may recommend ultrasound imaging to assess your baby's size, position, and overall well-being. Ultrasound measurements can provide additional information about your baby's growth trajectory.

3. Prenatal Testing:

A. Routine Screenings:

- Throughout your pregnancy, you'll undergo routine prenatal screenings and tests to monitor your baby's health and screen for potential complications. These may include blood tests, urine tests, ultrasound scans, and genetic screenings.

B. High-Risk Monitoring:

- If you have certain risk factors or medical conditions, such as gestational diabetes, hypertension, or a history of pregnancy complications, your healthcare provider may recommend additional monitoring and testing to ensure the best possible outcomes for you and your baby.

C. Non-Stress Test (NST):

- In the third trimester, your provider may perform non-stress tests (NSTs) to assess your baby's heart rate variability and response to movement. NSTs are often used to evaluate fetal well-being in high-risk pregnancies or when there are concerns about fetal distress.

4. Communicate with Your Healthcare Provider:

A. Open Communication:

- Be proactive about discussing any concerns or questions you have about your baby's health with your healthcare provider. Don't hesitate to reach out if you notice changes in fetal movements, have concerns about growth, or experience unusual symptoms.

B. Trust Your Instincts:

- As a mother, you know your baby best. Trust your instincts and seek medical attention if you ever feel that something isn't right. Your healthcare provider is there to support you and ensure the health and safety of both you and your baby.

C. Regular Prenatal Visits:

- Attend all scheduled prenatal visits and follow your provider's recommendations for monitoring your baby's health. These visits are essential for tracking your baby's growth, addressing any concerns, and ensuring a healthy pregnancy.

Chapter 6: The Second Trimester

What to Expect: Physical changes and symptom relief.

1. Morning Sickness and Nausea:

A. Symptoms:

- Nausea, vomiting, and sensitivity to certain smells are common symptoms, especially during the first trimester.

B. Relief Strategies:

- Eat small, frequent meals throughout the day to prevent hunger-induced nausea.
- Avoid strong smells and triggers that exacerbate nausea.
- Stay hydrated by sipping water or ginger tea.
- Try ginger supplements or candies to alleviate nausea.
- Consider acupressure wristbands or acupuncture for relief.

2. Fatigue:

A. Symptoms:

- Increased fatigue and feelings of exhaustion are common, especially during the first and third trimesters.

B. Relief Strategies:

- Prioritize rest and listen to your body's cues for additional sleep.
- Take short naps or breaks throughout the day to recharge.
- Stay active with gentle exercises like walking or prenatal yoga to boost energy levels.
- Maintain a balanced diet rich in iron and protein to combat fatigue.

3. Breast Tenderness:

A. Symptoms:

- Swelling, tenderness, and sensitivity in the breasts are common due to hormonal changes.

B. Relief Strategies:

- Wear a supportive and comfortable bra with good support.
- Consider wearing a sleep bra or soft sports bra for added comfort at night.
- Apply warm compresses or take warm baths to alleviate discomfort.
- Avoid caffeine and minimize salt intake to reduce breast swelling.

4. Frequent Urination:

A. Symptoms:

- Increased frequency of urination, especially during the first and third trimesters, due to pressure on the bladder from the growing uterus.

B. Relief Strategies:

- Stay hydrated but avoid excessive fluids close to bedtime to minimize nighttime bathroom trips.
- Practice pelvic floor exercises (Kegels) to strengthen bladder control.
- Empty your bladder completely each time you urinate to reduce the urge to go frequently.

5. Constipation:

A. Symptoms:

- Difficulty passing stools, infrequent bowel movements, and abdominal discomfort are common due to hormonal changes and pressure on the intestines.

B. Relief Strategies:

- Increase fiber intake with fruits, vegetables, whole grains, and legumes.
- Stay hydrated by drinking plenty of water throughout the day.
- Engage in regular physical activity to stimulate bowel movements.

- Consider safe over-the-counter laxatives or stool softeners if recommended by your healthcare provider.

6. Heartburn and Indigestion:

A. Symptoms:

- Burning sensation in the chest, stomach discomfort, and acid reflux are common due to hormonal changes and pressure on the stomach.

B. Relief Strategies:

- Eat smaller, more frequent meals to avoid overfilling the stomach.
- Avoid spicy, acidic, and greasy foods that trigger heartburn.
- Stay upright after eating to allow gravity to help prevent reflux.
- Consider antacids or other over-the-counter medications approved by your healthcare provider for relief.

Fetal Development: Milestones of the baby's growth.

1. Conception (Week 1-2):

A. Fertilization:

- Conception occurs when a sperm fertilizes an egg, forming a single cell called a zygote.
- The zygote contains the genetic material from both parents and begins to divide rapidly as it moves down the fallopian tube toward the uterus.

2. Embryonic Stage (Week 3-8):

A. Formation of Organs:

- During the embryonic stage, the major organs and body systems begin to form.
- The neural tube develops into the brain and spinal cord, and the heart begins to beat.
- Limb buds appear, and the basic structure of the arms, legs, fingers, and toes starts to form.

B. Growth Spurt:

- The embryo undergoes a period of rapid growth, increasing in size and complexity.
- Facial features, including eyes, ears, nose, and mouth, begin to take shape.

3. Fetal Stage (Week 9-Birth):

A. Organ Development:

- During the fetal stage, the focus shifts to further growth and refinement of organs and body structures.
- The fetus continues to develop and mature, with organs such as the lungs, liver, kidneys, and digestive system becoming fully functional.

B. Movement and Sensory Development:

- By the end of the first trimester, the fetus can move its limbs, open and close its fists, and make facial expressions.

- Sensory organs, including the eyes, ears, and taste buds, continue to develop, allowing the fetus to perceive light, sound, and taste.

C. Growth and Weight Gain:

- Throughout the second and third trimesters, the fetus experiences significant growth and weight gain.
- By the end of pregnancy, the average fetus weighs between 6-9 pounds and measures around 18-22 inches in length.

D. Fetal Movement:

- Fetal movements, also known as "quickening," become more pronounced and noticeable to the mother.
- The fetus may kick, stretch, and respond to stimuli, providing a tangible connection between mother and baby.

4. Final Trimester (Week 28-Birth):

A. Brain Development:

- The final trimester is crucial for brain development, including the growth of neurons, synapses, and myelin sheaths.
- The fetus demonstrates increased brain activity, preparing for life outside the womb.

B. Lung Maturation:

- The lungs continue to mature, producing surfactant, a substance that helps the air sacs inflate and prevents them from collapsing after birth.

- Surfactant production is essential for the baby's ability to breathe independently after delivery.

C. Positioning for Birth:

- In the weeks leading up to birth, the fetus typically settles into a head-down position in preparation for delivery.
- Some babies may remain in a breech or transverse position, requiring medical interventions or maneuvers to facilitate a safe delivery.

Managing Discomfort: Solutions for heartburn, back pain, and swelling.

1. Heartburn:

A. Dietary Adjustments:

- Eat smaller, more frequent meals throughout the day to prevent overloading your stomach.
- Avoid spicy, greasy, acidic, and fried foods that can trigger heartburn.
- Opt for lighter, more easily digestible meals and snacks.
- Stay upright after eating to allow gravity to help prevent acid reflux.

B. Lifestyle Modifications:

- Avoid lying down or bending over immediately after eating.
- Elevate the head of your bed with pillows to keep your upper body elevated while sleeping.
- Wear loose-fitting clothing to avoid putting pressure on your abdomen.

C. Over-the-Counter Remedies:

- Consider over-the-counter antacids or acid reducers approved by your healthcare provider for short-term relief of heartburn symptoms.
- Choose products that contain safe ingredients such as calcium carbonate or magnesium hydroxide.

2. Back Pain:

A. Proper Posture:

- Practice good posture by standing and sitting up straight, with your shoulders back and your pelvis tucked under.
- Use a supportive chair with good back support when sitting for extended periods.

B. Body Mechanics:

- Lift heavy objects with your legs, not your back, and avoid twisting your spine while lifting.
- Use proper body mechanics when getting in and out of bed or the car by rolling onto your side and pushing yourself up with your arms.

C. Exercise and Stretching:

- Engage in regular low-impact exercises such as walking, swimming, or prenatal yoga to strengthen your core and back muscles.
- Incorporate gentle stretching and flexibility exercises to improve mobility and reduce tension in your back.

D. Heat and Cold Therapy:

- Apply a warm compress or heating pad to your lower back to help relax tight muscles and alleviate pain.
- Alternatively, use a cold pack or ice pack wrapped in a cloth to reduce inflammation and numb soreness.

3. Swelling (Edema):

A. Stay Hydrated:

- Drink plenty of water throughout the day to stay hydrated and support healthy circulation.
- Limit your intake of caffeinated beverages, which can contribute to dehydration and exacerbate swelling.

B. Elevate Your Feet:

- Elevate your legs and feet whenever possible, especially after long periods of standing or sitting.
- Prop your feet up on a stool or ottoman to encourage fluid drainage and reduce swelling.

C. Compression Garments:

- Wear compression stockings or socks to provide gentle pressure and support to your legs and feet, helping to reduce swelling.
- Put on compression garments in the morning before swelling occurs for maximum effectiveness.

D. Regular Movement:

- Avoid prolonged periods of standing or sitting in the same position.

- Take short walks or perform gentle leg exercises throughout the day to promote circulation and reduce fluid retention.

Skin Changes: Dealing with stretch marks, acne, and pigmentation.

1. Stretch Marks:

A. Moisturize Regularly:

- Keep your skin hydrated by applying a moisturizing lotion or oil to areas prone to stretch marks, such as the abdomen, breasts, hips, and thighs.
- Look for products containing ingredients like cocoa butter, shea butter, vitamin E, or almond oil, which can help improve skin elasticity and reduce the appearance of stretch marks.

B. Gentle Massage:

- Incorporate gentle massage techniques into your skincare routine to promote circulation and encourage collagen production, which can help minimize the formation of stretch marks.
- Use circular motions to massage moisturizer or oil into the skin, focusing on areas with existing stretch marks or areas prone to stretching.

C. Wear Supportive Clothing:

- Choose supportive undergarments and clothing that provide adequate support to your growing belly and breasts, reducing the strain on your skin and minimizing the risk of stretch marks.
- Opt for maternity bras, supportive tank tops, and comfortable underwear with stretchy fabric and adjustable straps.

2. Acne:

A. Gentle Cleansing:

- Cleanse your skin twice daily with a mild, non-comedogenic cleanser to remove excess oil, dirt, and impurities without stripping the skin of its natural moisture.
- Avoid harsh or abrasive cleansers that can irritate the skin and exacerbate acne breakouts.

B. Spot Treatment:

- Use topical treatments containing ingredients like benzoyl peroxide, salicylic acid, or glycolic acid to target individual acne lesions and reduce inflammation.
- Be cautious when using acne treatments during pregnancy and consult with your healthcare provider to ensure they are safe for use during pregnancy.

C. Maintain a Healthy Lifestyle:

- Eat a balanced diet rich in fruits, vegetables, whole grains, and lean proteins to support overall skin health and reduce the risk of acne breakouts.
- Stay hydrated by drinking plenty of water throughout the day to flush out toxins and keep your skin hydrated from within.

3. Pigmentation (Melasma and Linea Nigra):

A. Sun Protection:

- Protect your skin from the sun's harmful UV rays by wearing broad-spectrum sunscreen with SPF 30 or higher every day, even on cloudy or overcast days.
- Wear protective clothing, such as wide-brimmed hats, sunglasses, and long sleeves, when outdoors to minimize sun exposure.

B. Gentle Exfoliation:

- Exfoliate your skin regularly with a gentle exfoliating scrub or chemical exfoliant containing ingredients like alpha hydroxy acids (AHAs) or beta hydroxy acids (BHAs) to promote cell turnover and reduce the appearance of pigmentation.

C. Makeup and Concealers:

- Use makeup and concealers to camouflage areas of pigmentation, such as melasma patches or linea nigra, if desired.
- Choose makeup products that are non-comedogenic and hypoallergenic to avoid clogging pores and exacerbating acne breakouts.

Chapter 7: The Third Trimester

Planning Ahead: Preparing for baby's arrival, from nurseries to maternity leave.

1. Creating a Nursery:

A. Design and Decor:

- Choose a theme or color scheme for the nursery that reflects your personal style and preferences.

- Select furniture items such as a crib, changing table, dresser, and rocking chair that are safe, functional, and aesthetically pleasing.
- Decorate the nursery with soft furnishings, wall art, and accessories to create a cozy and inviting space for your baby.

B. Organization and Storage:

- Invest in storage solutions such as bins, baskets, and shelves to keep baby essentials organized and easily accessible.
- Label storage containers for diapers, wipes, clothing, toys, and other baby items to streamline caregiving tasks.

C. Safety Measures:

- Babyproof the nursery by securing furniture to the wall, covering electrical outlets, and installing safety gates and window guards.
- Choose crib bedding, sleep sacks, and other sleep-related items that meet current safety standards to reduce the risk of Sudden Infant Death Syndrome (SIDS).

2. Arranging Maternity Leave:

A. Know Your Rights:

- Familiarize yourself with your employer's maternity leave policies, including the duration of leave, eligibility requirements, and benefits.
- Research federal and state laws governing maternity leave rights and protections, such as the Family and Medical Leave Act (FMLA) and the Pregnancy Discrimination Act (PDA).

B. Financial Planning:

- Assess your financial situation and budget to determine how much time you can afford to take off work without pay.
- Explore options for paid maternity leave, disability benefits, and other financial assistance programs available through your employer or government agencies.

C. Communicate with Your Employer:

- Notify your employer of your pregnancy and discuss your plans for maternity leave well in advance.
- Work with your employer to develop a maternity leave plan that meets both your needs and the needs of your employer.

3. Setting Up a Baby Registry:

A. Essential Items:

- Create a baby registry to compile a list of essential items you'll need for your baby, such as clothing, diapers, feeding supplies, and nursery gear.
- Include a variety of price points and items from different categories to accommodate the preferences and budgets of your friends and family members.

B. Research Products:

- Research baby products and brands to find high-quality, safe, and reliable items for your baby.
- Read reviews, seek recommendations from other parents, and consider factors such as safety, durability, and ease of use when selecting products for your registry.

C. Share Your Registry:

- Share your baby registry with friends and family members through online platforms, social media, or word of mouth to make it easy for them to find and purchase gifts for your baby.

4. Preparing Siblings and Pets:

A. Sibling Preparation:

- Involve older siblings in the preparations for the new baby by allowing them to help decorate the nursery, choose baby clothes, and select toys.
- Talk to older siblings about what to expect when the new baby arrives, including changes to routines and family dynamics.

B. Pet Adjustment:

- Gradually introduce pets to baby-related smells, sounds, and objects to help them acclimate to the upcoming changes.
- Establish boundaries and rules for interaction between pets and the new baby to ensure safety and positive experiences for everyone.

5. Self-Care and Support:

A. Rest and Relaxation:

- Prioritize self-care and rest during pregnancy to recharge and prepare for the demands of caring for a newborn.

- Practice relaxation techniques such as deep breathing, meditation, and gentle exercise to reduce stress and promote well-being.

B. Seek Support:

- Lean on your partner, family members, friends, and healthcare providers for emotional support, practical assistance, and guidance throughout your pregnancy journey.
- Join prenatal classes, support groups, or online communities to connect with other expectant parents and share experiences, advice, and resources.

Baby's Growth: Last stages of fetal development.

1. Organ Maturation:

A. Lung Development:

- In the third trimester, your baby's lungs continue to mature as they produce surfactant, a substance that helps the air sacs inflate and prevents them from collapsing after birth.
- Surfactant production is crucial for your baby's ability to breathe independently once they are born.

B. Brain and Nervous System:

- Your baby's brain undergoes rapid growth and development, with billions of neurons forming connections and pathways.
- The nervous system becomes more complex, allowing your baby to perceive and respond to stimuli, regulate body functions, and coordinate movements.

C. Digestive System:

- The digestive system matures as your baby's intestines develop the ability to absorb nutrients from amniotic fluid and prepare for the transition to breast milk or formula after birth.

2. Weight Gain and Growth:

A. Rapid Weight Gain:

- Your baby experiences significant weight gain during the third trimester, doubling or even tripling in size compared to earlier stages of pregnancy.
- Most of the weight gain during this period comes from the accumulation of fat stores, which provide insulation and energy reserves for your baby after birth.

B. Length and Size:

- Your baby's length and size continue to increase as they approach full-term gestation, with the average fetus measuring around 18-22 inches in length and weighing between 6-9 pounds by the end of pregnancy.

3. Fetal Movement and Positioning:

A. Increased Activity:

- As your baby grows larger and stronger, you may notice an increase in fetal movements, including kicks, rolls, and stretches.
- Fetal movements become more pronounced and noticeable as your baby explores their limited space in the uterus.

B. Positioning for Birth:

- In the weeks leading up to birth, your baby typically settles into a head-down position in preparation for delivery.
- Some babies may remain in a breech or transverse position, requiring medical interventions or maneuvers to facilitate a safe delivery.

4. Final Preparations for Birth:

A. Braxton Hicks Contractions:

- You may experience Braxton Hicks contractions, also known as "practice contractions," as your body prepares for labor.
- These contractions are usually irregular and mild, serving as a warm-up for the real contractions that occur during labor.

B. Engaging in the Pelvis:

- Towards the end of pregnancy, your baby's head may engage in your pelvis, also known as "lightening" or "dropping," as they get into position for birth.
- Engaging in the pelvis may relieve pressure on your diaphragm and allow you to breathe more easily, but it can also increase pressure on your bladder and pelvis.

Final Preparations: What to do in the last months of pregnancy.

1. Finalize Your Birth Plan:

A. Discuss Preferences:

- Review your birth plan with your healthcare provider and discuss your preferences for labor, delivery, and postpartum care.
- Consider factors such as pain management options, labor positions, and interventions to include in your plan.

B. Choose Your Support Team:

- Decide who will be present during labor and delivery, whether it's your partner, family members, or a doula.
- Communicate your preferences and expectations with your support team and ensure everyone is on the same page.

2. Attend Prenatal Classes:

A. Childbirth Education:

- Take childbirth education classes to learn about the stages of labor, coping techniques, and strategies for a positive birth experience.
- Attend breastfeeding classes to prepare for nursing and learn about proper latch, positioning, and newborn care.

B. Tour the Hospital or Birthing Center:

- Schedule a tour of the hospital or birthing center where you plan to deliver to familiarize yourself with the facilities and procedures.
- Ask questions about admission, labor and delivery rooms, and postpartum care services.

3. Prepare Your Home:

A. Set Up the Nursery:

- Complete the nursery setup by assembling furniture, decorating the room, and organizing baby essentials such as clothing, diapers, and bedding.
- Install safety measures such as baby gates, outlet covers, and furniture straps to childproof the nursery and other areas of your home.

B. Pack Your Hospital Bag:

- Pack a hospital bag with essential items for labor, delivery, and postpartum recovery, including comfortable clothing, toiletries, snacks, and entertainment.
- Include items for your partner and baby, such as a change of clothes, snacks, and a going-home outfit for the baby.

4. Stock Up on Essentials:

A. Baby Supplies:

- Stock up on newborn essentials such as diapers, wipes, diaper rash cream, and baby toiletries.
- Purchase baby gear such as a car seat, stroller, baby carrier, and breastfeeding supplies.

B. Postpartum Supplies:

- Gather postpartum supplies for your recovery, including sanitary pads, peri bottles, nursing bras, and comfortable underwear.
- Consider purchasing items to support breastfeeding, such as nursing pads, nipple cream, and a breastfeeding pillow.

5. Arrange Postpartum Support:

A. Support Network:

- Reach out to friends, family members, and neighbors for support during the postpartum period.
- Arrange for help with household chores, meal preparation, and childcare to ease the transition to parenthood.

B. Postpartum Care:

- Schedule postpartum check-ups with your healthcare provider to monitor your recovery and address any concerns.
- Seek out resources and support groups for new parents to connect with others and share experiences.

Signs of Labor: Recognizing pre-labor signs and Braxton Hicks contractions.

1. Pre-Labor Signs:

A. Lightening:

- In the weeks leading up to labor, you may experience "lightening" as your baby's head engages in your pelvis.
- This may result in decreased pressure on your diaphragm and increased pressure on your bladder, causing frequent urination.

B. Nesting Instinct:

- Many expectant mothers experience a surge of energy and an urge to prepare their home for the baby's arrival.
- This nesting instinct may involve organizing, cleaning, and completing last-minute tasks in anticipation of labor.

C. Cervical Changes:

- Your cervix may begin to soften, efface (thin out), and dilate (open up) in the days or weeks leading up to labor.
- Your healthcare provider may perform cervical checks during prenatal appointments to monitor these changes.

D. Bloody Show:

- A "bloody show" occurs when the mucus plug that seals the cervix during pregnancy is expelled, often accompanied by a small amount of blood.
- This may be a sign that your cervix is beginning to dilate in preparation for labor.

2. Braxton Hicks Contractions:

A. Timing:

- Braxton Hicks contractions are irregular and unpredictable, occurring at various times throughout the day.
- They may be more noticeable in the afternoon or evening but typically do not follow a regular pattern.

B. Intensity:

- Braxton Hicks contractions are usually mild and discomfort rather than painful.
- They may feel like a tightening or squeezing sensation in your abdomen, often described as feeling like a "practice contraction."

C. Relief:

- Braxton Hicks contractions typically subside with rest, hydration, or a change in position.
- They may lessen or disappear entirely after drinking water, taking a warm bath, or lying down on your left side.

D. Location:

- Braxton Hicks contractions may be felt in the front of your abdomen, as well as in your lower back or thighs.
- They may spread across your abdomen or be localized to one area.

Chapter 08: Labor and Delivery

Types of Delivery: Vaginal birth, C-section, and assisted delivery options.

1. Vaginal Birth:

A. Description:

- Vaginal birth, also known as natural birth or normal delivery, is the most common method of childbirth.
- It involves the baby passing through the birth canal (vagina) during labor and delivery.

B. Process:

- During labor, the cervix dilates (opens up) to allow the baby to descend through the birth canal.
- Contractions help push the baby downward, and the mother actively participates in the process by pushing during the second stage of labor.
- With proper support and pain management techniques, many women successfully deliver their babies vaginally.

C. Benefits:

- Vaginal birth is associated with shorter recovery times compared to C-section.
- It promotes early bonding between mother and baby and may reduce the risk of certain health complications for both.

2. Cesarean Section (C-Section):

A. Description:

- A Cesarean section, or C-section, is a surgical procedure in which the baby is delivered through an incision made in the mother's abdomen and uterus.

B. Indications:

- C-sections may be planned (elective) or performed as an emergency procedure in response to complications during labor.
- Common indications for C-section include fetal distress, breech presentation, placenta previa, and maternal health concerns.

C. Process:

- During a C-section, the mother is typically given anesthesia (either regional or general) to numb the lower half of her body or induce sleep.
- A surgical incision is made in the abdomen and uterus, and the baby is carefully delivered by the healthcare provider.
- The incisions are then closed with sutures or staples, and the mother is monitored closely during the recovery period.

D. Benefits:

- C-sections may be necessary to ensure the safety of the mother and baby in certain situations, such as fetal distress or complications with the placenta.
- They allow for controlled and expedited delivery in emergency situations, reducing the risk of adverse outcomes.

3. Assisted Delivery Options:

A. Forceps Delivery:

- Forceps delivery involves the use of specialized instruments (forceps) to gently guide the baby's head through the birth canal during labor.
- It may be recommended if the baby's position or progress is not optimal for a vaginal delivery, or if there are concerns about the baby's well-being.

B. Vacuum Extraction:

- Vacuum extraction, or vacuum-assisted delivery, utilizes a suction cup device (vacuum extractor) attached to the baby's head to assist with delivery.
- It is often used when there is a need to expedite delivery due to concerns about fetal distress or maternal exhaustion.

C. Indications and Considerations:

- Assisted delivery options are typically reserved for situations where vaginal delivery is preferred but additional support is needed to facilitate the process.
- They carry risks of complications, including maternal trauma, fetal injuries, and increased likelihood of episiotomy (surgical incision of the perineum).

Pain Relief: Epidurals, natural pain relief methods, and alternative options.

1. Epidurals:

A. Description:

- Epidural anesthesia is a common pain relief option for labor and delivery.
- It involves the administration of medication through a catheter placed in the lower back, near the spinal nerves that transmit pain signals from the uterus and birth canal.

B. Process:

- An anesthesiologist or nurse anesthetist administers the epidural medication, typically a combination of a local anesthetic and opioid analgesic.
- The epidural numbs the lower half of the body, providing pain relief while allowing the mother to remain awake and alert during childbirth.

C. Benefits:

- Epidurals provide effective pain relief for most women during labor and delivery, allowing them to rest and conserve energy for pushing.
- They can be adjusted to provide varying degrees of pain relief, depending on the mother's preferences and the progress of labor.

D. Considerations:

- Epidurals may be associated with potential side effects and complications, including low blood pressure, headache, nausea, and prolonged labor.
- It's essential to discuss the risks and benefits of epidural anesthesia with your healthcare provider and make an informed decision based on your individual circumstances.

2. Natural Pain Relief Methods:

A. Breathing Techniques:

- Deep breathing, relaxation, and mindfulness techniques can help manage pain and promote relaxation during contractions.
- Techniques such as Lamaze, Bradley, and Hypnobirthing focus on breathing exercises and relaxation strategies to cope with labor pain.

B. Movement and Positioning:

- Changing positions frequently, walking, rocking, and swaying can help alleviate discomfort and encourage progress during labor.

- Squatting, kneeling, and using a birthing ball or stool can also help open the pelvis and facilitate the descent of the baby.

C. Hydrotherapy:

- Immersion in water, such as taking a warm bath or shower, can provide soothing relief from labor pain and promote relaxation.
- Hydrotherapy may be available as an option for pain relief in some hospitals or birthing centers with access to birthing pools or tubs.

3. Alternative Pain Relief Options:

A. Acupuncture and Acupressure:

- Acupuncture involves the insertion of thin needles into specific points on the body to alleviate pain and promote relaxation.
- Acupressure applies pressure to these points using fingers or massage techniques to stimulate the body's natural pain-relieving mechanisms.

B. TENS (Transcutaneous Electrical Nerve Stimulation):

- TENS therapy involves the use of a small, battery-operated device that delivers mild electrical impulses to nerve pathways to reduce pain perception.
- TENS units may be used during labor to provide non-invasive pain relief and promote comfort.

C. Hypnotherapy:

- Hypnotherapy uses guided imagery, relaxation techniques, and suggestion to

> induce a state of deep relaxation and alter perceptions of pain.
> - Hypnosis during labor may help women manage pain, reduce anxiety, and enhance feelings of control and empowerment.

Birth Plan: Creating and discussing your birth plan with your healthcare provider.

1. Research Your Options:

A. Labor and Delivery Preferences:

- Research different labor and delivery options, including pain relief methods, birthing positions, and interventions such as fetal monitoring and episiotomy.
- Consider your preferences for pain management, including epidurals, natural pain relief techniques, and alternative options.

B. Postpartum Care Preferences:

- Think about your preferences for immediate postpartum care, including skin-to-skin contact, delayed cord clamping, and breastfeeding initiation.
- Consider any special requests or accommodations you may need, such as dietary restrictions, rooming-in with your baby, or support for breastfeeding.

2. Write Your Birth Plan:

A. Format:

- Use a clear and concise format to organize your birth plan, including sections for labor and delivery

preferences, pain relief options, and postpartum care preferences.
- Consider including bullet points or checkboxes to make it easy for your healthcare team to review and understand your preferences.

B. Include Your Preferences:

- Clearly state your preferences for labor and delivery, including your desired birth environment, birthing positions, and who you want to be present during labor.
- Outline your preferences for pain relief methods, such as epidurals, natural pain relief techniques, and alternative options like hydrotherapy or acupuncture.
- Specify your preferences for postpartum care, including immediate skin-to-skin contact, breastfeeding support, and delayed cord clamping.

3. Discuss Your Birth Plan with Your Healthcare Provider:

A. Schedule a Prenatal Appointment:

- Schedule a prenatal appointment with your healthcare provider to discuss your birth plan.
- Bring a copy of your birth plan to the appointment to review and discuss with your provider.

B. Ask Questions and Seek Clarification:

- Use the appointment as an opportunity to ask questions and seek clarification about any aspects of your birth plan.

- Discuss any concerns or preferences you have regarding labor, delivery, or postpartum care.

C. Be Open to Flexibility:

- Be open to discussing your birth plan with your healthcare provider and be willing to adapt your preferences based on medical necessity or unforeseen circumstances.
- Remember that the goal of your birth plan is to communicate your preferences and desires, but flexibility may be necessary depending on the circumstances of your labor and delivery.

4. Finalize Your Birth Plan:

A. Make Any Necessary Revisions:

- Make any necessary revisions to your birth plan based on your discussion with your healthcare provider.
- Ensure that your birth plan accurately reflects your preferences and desires for labor, delivery, and postpartum care.

B. Share Your Birth Plan:

- Share your finalized birth plan with your healthcare provider, birthing facility, and any other members of your birth team.
- Keep a copy of your birth plan with you during labor and delivery to reference and share with your healthcare team as needed.

Chapter 09: Postpartum Care

Physical Recovery: Healing after childbirth, dealing with postpartum bleeding and pain.

1. Postpartum Bleeding (Lochia):

A. Description:

- Lochia is the vaginal discharge that occurs after childbirth as the uterus sheds the lining that supported the pregnancy.
- It typically consists of blood, mucus, and tissue and can last for several weeks following delivery.

B. Types of Lochia:

- **Rubra:** Bright red bleeding that occurs in the first few days after childbirth, similar to a heavy menstrual period.
- **Serosa:** Pink or brownish discharge that occurs around days 4-10 postpartum as the bleeding slows down.
- **Alba:** Yellow or white discharge that occurs around days 10-14 postpartum as the bleeding tapers off.

C. Management:

- Use maternity pads or adult diapers to absorb the flow of lochia, changing them frequently as needed.
- Avoid using tampons or menstrual cups during the postpartum period to reduce the risk of infection.
- Monitor the color, amount, and odor of the discharge and contact your healthcare provider if you experience heavy bleeding, foul odor, or other concerning symptoms.

2. Postpartum Pain:

A. Perineal Pain:

- Perineal pain is common after vaginal childbirth, especially if you had an episiotomy or tearing during delivery.
- Use a peri-bottle filled with warm water to cleanse the perineal area after using the bathroom, and pat dry with a clean cloth.
- Sit on a cushion or donut-shaped pillow to relieve pressure on the perineum and promote healing.

B. Uterine Cramping:

- Uterine cramping is normal as the uterus contracts and returns to its pre-pregnancy size after childbirth.
- Use over-the-counter pain relievers such as acetaminophen (Tylenol) or ibuprofen (Advil, Motrin) to alleviate cramping discomfort, as recommended by your healthcare provider.
- Apply a heating pad or warm compress to the lower abdomen to help relax uterine muscles and reduce cramping.

C. Breast Engorgement:

- Breast engorgement, characterized by swollen, tender breasts, may occur as your milk comes in and your body adjusts to breastfeeding.
- Use cold compresses or cabbage leaves to reduce swelling and discomfort, and apply lanolin cream or nipple butter to soothe sore nipples.

- Nurse frequently or pump milk to relieve pressure and encourage milk flow, and ensure proper latching and positioning during breastfeeding to minimize discomfort.

3. Rest and Self-Care:

A. Prioritize Rest:

- Allow yourself time to rest and recover after childbirth, and accept help from family members, friends, or caregivers.
- Take short naps throughout the day when your baby sleeps, and prioritize sleep and relaxation whenever possible.

B. Hydration and Nutrition:

- Stay hydrated by drinking plenty of water throughout the day, and eat a balanced diet rich in nutrients to support your body's healing and recovery.
- Incorporate foods high in iron and fiber to replenish lost nutrients and promote healthy bowel movements.

C. Emotional Support:

- Seek emotional support from your partner, family members, or friends, and communicate openly about your feelings and experiences.
- Consider joining a support group for new mothers or seeking counseling or therapy if you're struggling with postpartum emotions or mood changes.

Mental Health: Recognizing and treating postpartum depression.

1. Recognizing Signs and Symptoms:

A. Persistent Sadness or Hopelessness:

- Feelings of sadness, emptiness, or hopelessness that persist for more than two weeks after childbirth.

B. Loss of Interest or Pleasure:

- Loss of interest or enjoyment in activities that were once pleasurable, including activities related to caring for the baby.

C. Irritability or Mood Swings:

- Increased irritability, mood swings, or agitation, even in situations that wouldn't typically trigger such emotions.

D. Fatigue or Loss of Energy:

- Persistent fatigue or loss of energy, even after getting adequate rest or sleep.

E. Changes in Appetite or Sleep Patterns:

- Changes in appetite, including loss of appetite or overeating, as well as changes in sleep patterns, such as insomnia or excessive sleeping.

F. Difficulty Bonding with the Baby:

- Difficulty bonding with the baby or feeling disconnected from the baby, despite attempts to engage in caregiving activities.

G. Feelings of Guilt or Worthlessness:

- Feelings of guilt, worthlessness, or self-blame, often accompanied by intrusive or negative thoughts.

H. Thoughts of Self-Harm or Suicidal Ideation:

- Thoughts of self-harm, suicide, or harming the baby, as well as feelings of being a burden or wanting to escape.

2. Seeking Help and Treatment:

A. Talk to Your Healthcare Provider:

- If you experience any signs or symptoms of postpartum depression, it's essential to talk to your healthcare provider as soon as possible.
- Your healthcare provider can assess your symptoms, provide support and guidance, and recommend appropriate treatment options.

B. Therapy and Counseling:

- Therapy, such as cognitive-behavioral therapy (CBT) or interpersonal therapy (IPT), can be highly effective in treating postpartum depression.
- Counseling sessions provide a safe space to explore your feelings, develop coping strategies, and address underlying issues contributing to PPD.

C. Medication:

- In some cases, antidepressant medication may be prescribed to help manage symptoms of postpartum depression.
- Selective serotonin reuptake inhibitors (SSRIs) are often the first-line treatment for PPD and are generally considered safe for breastfeeding mothers.

D. Support Groups:

- Joining a support group for mothers with postpartum depression can provide valuable peer support, validation, and encouragement.
- Support groups offer an opportunity to share experiences, learn from others, and reduce feelings of isolation and stigma associated with PPD.

E. Self-Care Strategies:

- Prioritize self-care activities such as adequate rest, regular exercise, healthy nutrition, and engaging in activities that promote relaxation and well-being.
- Set realistic expectations for yourself and ask for help from family members, friends, or support networks when needed.

3. Involving Your Support Network:

A. Partner and Family Support:

- Involve your partner and family members in your treatment plan and communicate openly about your feelings and needs.
- Encourage your partner to participate in therapy sessions or support group meetings to gain a better understanding of postpartum depression and how to provide support.

B. Childcare Assistance:

- Seek help with childcare responsibilities from family members, friends, or childcare providers to give yourself time to focus on self-care and treatment.

Self-care Tips: Taking care of your body and mind after delivery.

1. Rest and Recovery:

A. Prioritize Sleep:

- Aim to get as much rest as possible, even if it means taking short naps throughout the day when your baby sleeps.
- Consider co-sleeping or room-sharing with your baby to make nighttime feedings and comforting easier.

B. Accept Help:

- Don't hesitate to accept help from family members, friends, or caregivers to lighten your workload and give yourself time to rest and recover.
- Delegate household chores, meal preparation, and childcare responsibilities to others whenever possible.

2. Nutrition and Hydration:

A. Eat Nutrient-Rich Foods:

- Focus on eating a balanced diet rich in fruits, vegetables, lean proteins, whole grains, and healthy fats to support your body's healing and recovery.
- Incorporate foods high in iron, calcium, and fiber to replenish lost nutrients and promote optimal health.

B. Stay Hydrated:

- Drink plenty of water throughout the day to stay hydrated, especially if you're breastfeeding.
- Limit caffeinated and sugary beverages and opt for water, herbal teas, and fruit-infused water instead.

3. Physical Care:

A. Practice Gentle Exercise:

- Engage in gentle postpartum exercises such as walking, stretching, pelvic floor exercises (Kegels), and postpartum yoga to promote circulation, strength, and flexibility.
- Start slowly and gradually increase the intensity and duration of your workouts as your body heals.

B. Practice Perineal Care:

- Use a peri-bottle filled with warm water to cleanse the perineal area after using the bathroom, and pat dry with a clean cloth.
- Take sitz baths with warm water and Epsom salts to soothe perineal discomfort and promote healing.

4. Emotional Well-Being:

A. Connect with Others:

- Seek support from your partner, family members, friends, or support groups for new mothers to share your experiences, feelings, and concerns.

- Surround yourself with positive and understanding individuals who can offer empathy, encouragement, and practical assistance.

B. Prioritize Self-Care:

- Make time for self-care activities that promote relaxation, stress relief, and emotional well-being.
- Engage in activities that bring you joy and fulfillment, such as reading, journaling, listening to music, or practicing mindfulness and meditation.

5. Seek Professional Support:

A. Schedule Regular Check-Ups:

- Attend postpartum check-ups with your healthcare provider to monitor your physical and emotional health, address any concerns, and ensure optimal recovery.

B. Seek Therapy or Counseling:

- If you're struggling with postpartum emotions, mood changes, or mental health issues such as postpartum depression or anxiety, don't hesitate to seek therapy or counseling.
- Therapy sessions provide a safe and supportive space to explore your feelings, develop coping strategies, and receive guidance and support from a trained professional.

Chapter 10: Breastfeeding

Benefits: Why breastfeeding is beneficial for both mother and baby.

Benefits for the Baby:

1. Optimal Nutrition:

- Breast milk is uniquely tailored to meet the nutritional needs of infants, providing essential nutrients, antibodies, and immune factors that support growth and development.

2. Immune Protection:

- Breast milk contains antibodies and immune factors that help protect babies from infections, illnesses, and diseases, reducing the risk of respiratory infections, ear infections, gastrointestinal infections, and other illnesses.

3. Reduced Risk of Chronic Conditions:

- Breastfeeding is associated with a reduced risk of chronic conditions and diseases later in life, including obesity, type 2 diabetes, asthma, allergies, and certain types of cancer.

4. Cognitive Development:

- Breastfeeding has been linked to improved cognitive development and higher IQ scores in children, likely due to the presence of essential fatty acids and other nutrients in breast milk.

5. Digestive Health:

- Breast milk is easily digested and may help prevent digestive issues such as constipation, diarrhea, and gastroesophageal reflux in infants.

6. Emotional Bonding:

- Breastfeeding promotes a strong emotional bond between mother and baby, fostering feelings of security, comfort, and attachment that contribute to healthy emotional development.

Benefits for the Mother:

1. Faster Postpartum Recovery:

- Breastfeeding stimulates the release of hormones that help the uterus contract and return to its pre-pregnancy size, leading to faster postpartum recovery and reduced postpartum bleeding.

2. Weight Loss:

- Breastfeeding burns calories and helps mothers lose pregnancy weight more quickly, promoting gradual weight loss and improved body composition.

3. Reduced Risk of Breast and Ovarian Cancer:

- Breastfeeding is associated with a reduced risk of breast and ovarian cancer in mothers, particularly when practiced for an extended duration.

4. Hormonal Regulation:

- Breastfeeding promotes hormonal balance and may help regulate menstrual cycles,

delaying the return of ovulation and
fertility in some women.

5. Emotional Well-Being:

- Breastfeeding releases hormones such as oxytocin, which
  promotes feelings of relaxation, bonding, and well-being in
  mothers, reducing the risk of postpartum depression and
  anxiety.

6. Cost Savings:

- Breastfeeding is cost-effective and convenient, eliminating
  the need for formula feeding supplies and reducing
  healthcare costs associated with infant illnesses and
  hospitalizations.

Techniques: How to latch, different breastfeeding positions,
and dealing with common challenges.

1. Achieving a Proper Latch:

A. Positioning:

- Sit or recline in a comfortable chair with good back support,
  and use pillows or cushions to support your arms and baby.
- Bring your baby to breast level, tummy to tummy, and ensure
  that their head, neck, and body are aligned in a straight line.

B. Latching Technique:

- Wait for your baby to open their mouth wide, like a yawn,
  before bringing them to the breast.
- Aim your nipple toward the roof of your baby's mouth and
  guide them to latch onto the areola (the dark area
  surrounding the nipple) rather than just the nipple itself.

- Ensure that your baby's lips are flanged outward (turned outward) and their chin is pressed into your breast, with their nose clear for breathing.

C. Signs of a Good Latch:

- Your baby's mouth covers a large portion of the areola, and their lips form a tight seal around the breast.
- You may feel a gentle tugging or pulling sensation, but breastfeeding should not be painful.
- Your baby's cheeks should appear rounded and full during feeding.

2. Different Breastfeeding Positions:

A. Cradle Hold:

- Support your baby's head with one hand and their body with your forearm, bringing them to your breast with their head resting in the crook of your arm.
- This position is ideal for newborns and younger babies and allows for eye contact and bonding.

B. Football Hold:

- Position your baby at your side with their legs tucked under your arm, like a football, and their head supported by your hand.
- This position is useful for mothers recovering from a cesarean section or with large breasts, as it provides better visibility and control.

C. Side-Lying Position:

- Lie on your side with your baby facing you, and bring them close to your breast for feeding.
- This position is comfortable for nighttime feedings or when you need to rest, allowing you to relax while nursing.

3. Dealing with Common Challenges:

A. Engorgement:

- Apply warm compresses or take a warm shower to encourage milk flow and relieve discomfort.
- Express a small amount of milk by hand or pump before feeding to soften the breast and make latching easier for your baby.

B. Sore Nipples:

- Ensure a proper latch to minimize friction and rubbing on the nipples.
- Apply lanolin cream or purified lanolin after each feeding to soothe and protect sore nipples.

C. Low Milk Supply:

- Nurse frequently and on demand to stimulate milk production and maintain a healthy milk supply.
- Stay hydrated, eat a balanced diet, and get adequate rest to support milk production.

D. Breastfeeding Pain:

- Address any underlying issues such as tongue tie or thrush that may be causing pain during breastfeeding.

- Seek support from a lactation consultant or healthcare provider to assess latch and positioning and provide guidance on pain management techniques.

Support: Resources and support groups for breastfeeding mothers.

1. Lactation Consultants:

A. What They Do:

- Lactation consultants are trained professionals who specialize in breastfeeding support and education.
- They can assess latch and positioning, provide guidance on breastfeeding techniques, and offer solutions to common breastfeeding challenges.

B. How to Find One:

- Ask your healthcare provider, pediatrician, or hospital for a referral to a certified lactation consultant.
- Many hospitals and birthing centers have lactation consultants on staff who can provide support during your hospital stay and after discharge.

2. La Leche League International (LLLI):

A. Overview:

- La Leche League International is a nonprofit organization dedicated to promoting breastfeeding and providing support to breastfeeding mothers worldwide.
- They offer resources, educational materials, and support group meetings led by trained leaders.

B. How to Get Involved:

- Visit the La Leche League International website to find a local chapter or support group meeting in your area.
- Attend meetings to connect with other breastfeeding mothers, share experiences, and receive guidance and encouragement from trained leaders.

3. Breastfeeding Support Hotlines:

A. Overview:

- Breastfeeding support hotlines provide free, confidential support and information to breastfeeding mothers over the phone.
- Trained volunteers or lactation consultants are available to answer questions, address concerns, and provide guidance on breastfeeding issues.

B. How to Access:

- Check with your local breastfeeding support organizations or healthcare providers to inquire about breastfeeding support hotlines available in your area.
- Save hotline numbers in your phone or write them down for easy access when you need assistance.

4. Online Communities and Forums:

A. Overview:

- Online communities and forums provide a platform for breastfeeding mothers to connect, share experiences, and seek advice from peers.
- Websites and social media platforms host groups and forums dedicated to breastfeeding support, where mothers can ask questions, offer support, and share resources.

B. How to Join:

- Search for breastfeeding support groups on social media platforms like Facebook or forums dedicated to parenting and breastfeeding.
- Join online communities that resonate with your interests and values, and participate in discussions, ask questions, and offer support to other members.

5. Local Support Groups:

A. Overview:

- Many communities offer local support groups for breastfeeding mothers, facilitated by healthcare providers, lactation consultants, or trained volunteers.
- These groups provide opportunities for mothers to connect face-to-face, share experiences, and receive support and guidance in a supportive environment.

B. How to Find One:

- Inquire with your healthcare provider, hospital, or community center about local breastfeeding support groups or mom-to-mom groups in your area.

- Attend meetings or gatherings to meet other breastfeeding mothers and build a network of support within your community.

Chapter 11: Bottle Feeding

Choosing Formula: Types of formula and how to choose the best one.

1. Types of Formula:

A. Cow's Milk-Based Formula:

- Most infant formulas are made from cow's milk that has been modified to resemble breast milk in composition.
- Cow's milk-based formula is suitable for the majority of healthy, full-term infants and provides essential nutrients such as protein, carbohydrates, fats, vitamins, and minerals.

B. Soy-Based Formula:

- Soy-based formula is made from soy protein and is suitable for babies who are allergic to cow's milk protein or have lactose intolerance.
- It provides a plant-based alternative to cow's milk-based formula and is fortified with essential nutrients to support healthy growth and development.

C. Hydrolyzed Formula:

- Hydrolyzed formula is specially designed for babies with cow's milk protein allergy or difficulty digesting intact proteins.
- It contains proteins that have been broken down (hydrolyzed) into smaller, more easily digestible

fragments, reducing the risk of allergic reactions and digestive issues.

D. Specialized Formulas:

- Specialized formulas are available for babies with specific dietary or medical needs, such as premature infants, babies with reflux or colic, or those with metabolic disorders.
- These formulas may contain additional nutrients, supplements, or modifications to address unique nutritional requirements or health concerns.

2. Factors to Consider:

A. Baby's Age and Developmental Stage:

- Choose a formula that is appropriate for your baby's age and developmental stage, as nutritional needs may vary during infancy.
- Infant formulas are available in different formulations for newborns, older infants, and toddlers, with varying nutrient compositions to support growth and development.

B. Allergies and Sensitivities:

- Consider any known allergies or sensitivities your baby may have when selecting a formula.
- If your baby has a family history of allergies or allergic reactions to cow's milk protein, you may opt for a soy-based or hydrolyzed formula to reduce the risk of allergic reactions.

C. Nutritional Composition:

- Review the nutritional composition of different formulas to ensure they meet your baby's dietary needs.
- Look for formulas that are fortified with essential nutrients such as iron, calcium, vitamin D, and omega-3 fatty acids to support healthy growth and development.

D. Preparation and Convenience:

- Consider factors such as ease of preparation, storage, and convenience when choosing a formula.
- Some formulas come in ready-to-feed liquid form, while others require mixing with water or powder reconstitution, so choose a format that fits your lifestyle and preferences.

3. Consultation with Healthcare Providers:

A. Pediatrician or Healthcare Provider:

- Consult with your pediatrician or healthcare provider before introducing formula to your baby, especially if you have any concerns or questions about their nutritional needs or feeding preferences.
- Your healthcare provider can offer guidance and recommendations based on your baby's individual needs and circumstances.

B. Lactation Consultant or Registered Dietitian:

- If you're transitioning from breastfeeding to formula feeding or have specific questions about infant nutrition, consider seeking guidance from a lactation consultant or registered dietitian who specializes in pediatric nutrition.

- These professionals can provide personalized advice and support to help you make informed decisions about formula feeding and infant nutrition.

Feeding Schedule: Creating a feeding routine for your baby.

1. Newborn Feeding Patterns:

A. On-Demand Feeding:

- In the early weeks, newborns typically feed on-demand, meaning they signal hunger cues (rooting, sucking on fists, crying) when they're hungry, rather than adhering to a strict schedule.
- Feed your baby whenever they show signs of hunger, which may occur every 2-3 hours or more frequently, including during the night.

B. Cluster Feeding:

- Cluster feeding refers to periods when your baby feeds more frequently or for longer durations, often in the evening hours.
- During cluster feeding sessions, offer your baby frequent, smaller feedings to satisfy their hunger and help increase milk supply.

2. Establishing a Feeding Routine:

A. Frequency of Feedings:

- As your baby grows and matures, you can gradually establish a more structured feeding routine, with feedings spaced out approximately every 2-3 hours during the day.

- Aim for 8-12 feedings per 24-hour period, adjusting the frequency based on your baby's hunger cues and individual needs.

B. Duration of Feedings:

- Encourage your baby to nurse or bottle-feed until they appear satisfied and content, rather than limiting feedings based on a predetermined timeframe.
- Allow your baby to feed at their own pace, pausing for burping or breaks as needed during feedings.

3. Daytime vs. Nighttime Feedings:

A. Daytime Feedings:

- During the day, aim for more wakeful, alert feedings with opportunities for interaction and bonding between you and your baby.
- Offer feedings in a well-lit, comfortable environment, and take breaks for diaper changes, cuddling, and playtime between feedings.

B. Nighttime Feedings:

- While newborns may still require nighttime feedings, aim to keep nighttime feedings calm, quiet, and low-stimulation to promote restful sleep for both you and your baby.
- Keep the lights dimmed, minimize noise and distractions, and focus on soothing your baby back to sleep after feedings.

4. Responsive Feeding:

A. Reading Hunger Cues:

- Pay attention to your baby's hunger cues and feeding cues, such as rooting, sucking motions, hand-to-mouth movements, and increased alertness.
- Respond promptly to your baby's cues by offering feedings when they're hungry and stopping when they show signs of fullness.

B. Flexibility and Adaptation:

- Be flexible and adaptable with your feeding schedule, especially during growth spurts, developmental leaps, or times of illness when your baby may need more frequent feedings or extra comfort.

5. Keeping Track of Feedings:

A. Feeding Log:

- Consider keeping a feeding log or journal to track your baby's feeding times, durations, and diaper output.
- A feeding log can help you identify feeding patterns, monitor your baby's growth and development, and provide valuable information for discussions with healthcare providers.

B. Using Feeding Apps:

- There are various smartphone apps available that can help you track feedings, diaper changes, sleep patterns, and other aspects of your baby's daily routine.

- Look for apps with user-friendly interfaces and customizable features to meet your specific tracking needs and preferences.

Sterilization and Hygiene: Keeping bottles and feeding equipment clean.

1. Cleaning Bottles and Accessories:

A. Hand Washing:

- Wash bottles, nipples, rings, caps, and other feeding accessories thoroughly with warm, soapy water immediately after each use.
- Use a bottle brush to clean the inside of bottles and nipples, ensuring that all residue and milk deposits are removed.

B. Rinse Thoroughly:

- Rinse bottles and accessories with clean, running water to remove soap residue and any remaining debris.
- Pay special attention to crevices, seams, and bottle nipples to ensure thorough rinsing.

C. Air Dry:

- Allow bottles and accessories to air dry on a clean drying rack or surface, avoiding the use of towels or cloths that may harbor bacteria.
- Ensure that bottles are completely dry before assembling or storing to prevent the growth of mold and bacteria.

2. Sterilization Methods:

A. Boiling:

- Boil bottles, nipples, and accessories in a pot of water for at least 5 minutes to sterilize them effectively.
- Use a clean pair of tongs to remove items from the boiling water and allow them to cool before use.

B. Steam Sterilization:

- Use an electric steam sterilizer or microwave steam sterilizing bags designed for baby bottles and accessories.
- Follow manufacturer instructions for proper use and duration of steam sterilization cycles.

C. Dishwasher Sterilization:

- If dishwasher-safe, place bottles, nipples, and accessories in the dishwasher and run them through a hot water and high-temperature cycle.
- Ensure that items are arranged securely in the dishwasher to prevent them from moving around or falling during the cycle.

3. Storage and Handling:

A. Store in a Clean Environment:

- Store sterilized bottles and feeding equipment in a clean, dry environment away from dust, dirt, and other contaminants.

- Use covered containers or storage bags to protect items from exposure to airborne particles and pests.

B. Avoid Cross-Contamination:

- Handle sterilized bottles and accessories with clean hands and avoid touching the inside surfaces that will come into contact with milk or formula.
- Use separate storage areas or compartments for sterilized and unsterilized items to prevent cross-contamination.

C. Regular Inspection:

- Inspect bottles, nipples, and accessories regularly for signs of wear, damage, or deterioration.
- Discard any items that show signs of damage, such as cracks, chips, or discoloration, as they may harbor bacteria or pose a choking hazard to your baby.

4. Additional Tips:

A. Clean Preparation Area:

- Maintain a clean and sanitized preparation area for handling bottles, formula, and feeding equipment.
- Wipe down countertops, surfaces, and utensils with disinfectant wipes or a solution of water and bleach to minimize the risk of contamination.

B. Breast Pump Hygiene:

- If using a breast pump, follow manufacturer instructions for cleaning and sterilizing pump parts after each use.
- Store pump parts in a clean, dry container or bag between uses to prevent contamination.

Chapter 12: Newborn Care

First Days: What to expect in the first days and weeks with your newborn.

1. Initial Bonding:

A. Skin-to-Skin Contact:

- Encourage bonding and attachment with your newborn through skin-to-skin contact, which promotes warmth, comfort, and emotional connection.
- Hold your baby against your bare chest, cuddle them close, and engage in gentle touch, eye contact, and soothing sounds.

B. Breastfeeding or Bottle-Feeding:

- Establish feeding routines and practices, whether breastfeeding or bottle-feeding, to nourish your baby and promote bonding.
- Allow plenty of time for feeding sessions, taking breaks for burping, cuddling, and bonding during and after feedings.

2. Newborn Care:

A. Diaper Changes:

- Expect frequent diaper changes, as newborns typically urinate and pass stools several times a day.

- Keep a supply of diapers, wipes, and diaper rash cream handy, and change your baby's diaper promptly whenever it's wet or soiled.

B. Umbilical Cord Care:

- Follow guidelines for caring for your baby's umbilical cord stump, keeping it clean and dry until it falls off naturally within the first few weeks.
- Avoid submerging your baby in water until the umbilical cord stump has healed and fallen off to prevent infection.

3. Sleep Patterns:

A. Irregular Sleep Patterns:

- Expect your newborn to sleep for short periods throughout the day and night, with frequent awakenings for feeding, diaper changes, and comfort.
- Newborn sleep patterns are often irregular and may vary from one day to the next, so be prepared for interrupted sleep and daytime naps.

B. Safe Sleep Practices:

- Create a safe sleep environment for your baby by placing them on their back to sleep in a crib or bassinet with a firm mattress and tight-fitting sheet.
- Avoid using pillows, blankets, crib bumpers, or soft bedding that may pose a suffocation risk to your baby.

4. Physical Development:

A. Newborn Reflexes:

- Notice your baby's reflexes and responses, such as rooting, sucking, grasping, and startle reflexes, which are essential for survival and development.
- Observe your baby's motor skills and milestones as they learn to lift their head, track objects with their eyes, and explore their surroundings.

B. Growth and Weight Gain:

- Monitor your baby's growth and weight gain through regular check-ups with your pediatrician or healthcare provider.
- Expect your baby to lose a small amount of weight in the first days after birth, followed by steady weight gain as they adjust to feeding and grow.

5. Emotional Adjustment:

A. Hormonal Changes:

- Be aware of hormonal changes and emotional fluctuations that may occur in the first days and weeks after childbirth, known as the "baby blues."
- It's normal to experience mood swings, feelings of sadness, anxiety, or overwhelm as you navigate the challenges and joys of parenthood.

B. Support Network:

- Seek support from your partner, family members, friends, and healthcare providers as you adjust to parenthood and care for your newborn.
- Don't hesitate to ask for help, share your feelings, and lean on your support network for emotional support, guidance, and practical assistance.

Basic Care: Bathing, diapering, and dressing your baby.

1. Bathing Your Baby:

A. Frequency:

- Newborns typically only need to be bathed 2-3 times per week to keep their skin clean and healthy.
- In the early days after birth, you can sponge bathe your baby until their umbilical cord stump falls off.

B. Supplies:

- Gather all necessary supplies before bathing your baby, including a basin of warm water, mild baby soap or cleanser, soft washcloths, towels, clean clothes, and any other bath accessories.

C. Technique:

- Support your baby's head and neck with one hand while gently washing their body with the other hand.
- Use mild soap or cleanser to wash your baby's face, body, and hair, rinsing thoroughly with warm water.
- Pay special attention to folds and creases, such as behind the ears, under the arms, and in diaper areas, to prevent the buildup of dirt and moisture.

D. Safety:

- Never leave your baby unattended in the bath, even for a moment, as drowning can occur in as little as an inch of water.
- Keep the water temperature warm, but not too hot, to prevent scalding or burns.

2. Diapering Your Baby:

A. Supplies:

- Have all diapering supplies within reach before beginning, including diapers, wipes, diaper rash cream, and a clean changing surface.

B. Technique:

- Lay your baby on their back on a clean, flat surface, such as a changing table or bed, with a waterproof pad or towel underneath.
- Remove the dirty diaper, wiping your baby's bottom gently with baby wipes from front to back.
- Apply diaper rash cream if needed, then place a clean diaper under your baby and fasten securely.

C. Preventing Diaper Rash:

- Change your baby's diaper promptly whenever it's wet or soiled to prevent diaper rash and skin irritation.
- Allow your baby's skin to air dry between diaper changes, and consider using a barrier cream to protect against moisture and irritation.

3. Dressing Your Baby:

A. Comfort and Safety:

- Choose soft, comfortable clothing made from breathable fabrics such as cotton to keep your baby cool and comfortable.
- Dress your baby in layers to accommodate changes in temperature, and avoid overdressing to prevent overheating.

B. Technique:

- Lay your baby on a flat surface or hold them securely on your lap while dressing.
- Dress your baby from the top down, starting with a clean undershirt or onesie, followed by pants or a sleeper, and finishing with socks or booties if needed.

C. Avoiding Overstimulation:

- Keep dressing sessions calm and soothing, avoiding excessive handling or stimulation that may upset or overstimulate your baby.
- Provide gentle reassurance and soothing sounds or lullabies to help your baby feel secure and comforted during dressing.

Chapter 13: Work and Pregnancy

Balancing Work and Pregnancy: Tips for managing work during pregnancy.

1. Communicate with Your Employer:

A. Inform Early: Notify your employer about your pregnancy as soon as you feel comfortable, especially if you anticipate needing accommodations or adjustments to your workload.

B. Discuss Needs: Discuss any necessary accommodations or modifications to your job duties with your employer, such as ergonomic changes, flexible scheduling, or time off for prenatal appointments.

C. Know Your Rights: Familiarize yourself with your rights under the law, including protections provided by the Family and Medical Leave Act (FMLA) or the Pregnancy Discrimination Act (PDA), and advocate for yourself if needed.

2. Prioritize Self-Care:

A. Listen to Your Body: Pay attention to your body's signals and adjust your workload or schedule as needed to accommodate fatigue, nausea, or other pregnancy symptoms.

B. Take Breaks: Incorporate regular breaks into your workday to rest, stretch, and recharge, especially if you have a desk job or spend long hours sitting.

C. Stay Hydrated: Drink plenty of water throughout the day to stay hydrated and maintain energy levels, especially if you're experiencing increased thirst due to pregnancy.

3. Manage Stress:

A. Set Boundaries: Establish boundaries between work and personal life to prevent burnout and maintain a healthy work-life balance.

B. Delegate Tasks: Delegate tasks or responsibilities when possible to lighten your workload and reduce stress, both at work and at home.

C. Practice Relaxation Techniques: Incorporate stress-reduction techniques such as deep breathing, meditation, or gentle exercise into your daily routine to promote relaxation and mental well-being.

4. Stay Organized:

A. Plan Ahead: Stay organized by prioritizing tasks, setting realistic goals, and planning ahead for deadlines or projects that may coincide with your due date.

B. Create To-Do Lists: Use to-do lists or scheduling tools to keep track of important tasks, appointments, and deadlines, and break larger projects into smaller, manageable steps.

C. Communicate with Colleagues: Keep open lines of communication with your colleagues or supervisors about your workload, availability, and any adjustments needed during your pregnancy.

5. Seek Support:

A. Lean on Your Support Network: Reach out to your partner, family members, friends, or coworkers for emotional support, practical assistance, or advice when needed.

B. Join Support Groups: Consider joining a pregnancy support group or online community to connect with other expectant parents, share experiences, and receive encouragement and advice.
C. Talk to Healthcare Providers: Discuss any concerns or challenges related to work and pregnancy with your healthcare provider, who can offer guidance and support tailored to your individual needs.

Maternity Leave: Understanding your rights and planning for time off.

1. Know Your Rights:

A. Familiarize Yourself with Company Policies: Review your employer's maternity leave policies, including provisions for paid or unpaid leave, duration, eligibility requirements, and benefits such as continued health insurance coverage.
B. Understand Legal Protections: Understand your rights under federal and state laws, such as the Family and Medical Leave Act (FMLA) or the Pregnancy Discrimination Act (PDA), which provide certain protections for pregnant employees, including job protection and unpaid leave.
C. Consult Human Resources: If you have questions or concerns about your maternity leave entitlements or rights, consult with your company's human resources department or seek guidance from legal resources specializing in employment law.

2. Plan Ahead:

A. Determine Timing: Decide when you plan to start your maternity leave based on your due date, health considerations, and personal preferences. Some women choose to begin leave a few weeks before their due date, while others prefer to work as long as possible and save leave for after the baby arrives.

B. Review Finances: Assess your financial situation and budget to determine how much time off you can afford to take and whether you need to supplement unpaid leave with savings, disability insurance, or other sources of income.

C. Coordinate with Partner: If your partner also plans to take time off to care for the baby, coordinate your leave schedules and discuss how to divide caregiving responsibilities during your absence from work.

3. Communicate with Your Employer:

A. Provide Advance Notice: Notify your employer of your pregnancy and your intention to take maternity leave as soon as possible, following company procedures for requesting leave and providing necessary documentation.

B. Discuss Leave Arrangements: Meet with your supervisor or HR representative to discuss the details of your maternity leave, including the duration, anticipated return date, any special accommodations needed, and plans for transitioning your workload during your absence.

C. Stay in Touch: Stay in communication with your employer and colleagues during your leave, if possible, to stay informed about any important updates or changes in the workplace and facilitate a smooth return to work.

4. Plan for Return:

A. Arrange Childcare: Make arrangements for childcare or caregiving support well in advance of your return to work, whether it's enrolling your baby in daycare, hiring a nanny, or arranging care with family members or friends.

B. Ease into Work: Consider negotiating a gradual return to work schedule, such as part-time hours or a phased return, to ease the transition and allow time to adjust to your new role as a working parent.

C. Prioritize Self-Care: Be gentle with yourself as you transition back to work, and prioritize self-care to manage stress and maintain balance between work and family responsibilities.

Returning to Work: Preparing for the transition back to work after maternity leave.

1. Plan Ahead:

A. Determine Return Date: Decide on your return-to-work date in advance, considering factors such as your baby's age, childcare arrangements, and personal readiness.

B. Arrange Childcare: Research and secure childcare arrangements well in advance, whether it's daycare, a nanny, or family members. Visit childcare facilities, interview caregivers, and ensure you feel comfortable with your choice.

C. Set Up Logistics: Organize practical aspects of your return, such as transportation, meal planning, and scheduling, to streamline your daily routine and reduce stress during the transition.

2. Communicate with Your Employer:

A. Stay in Touch: Maintain open lines of communication with your employer and colleagues during your maternity leave, staying informed about any updates or changes in the workplace.

B. Discuss Work Arrangements: Have a conversation with your supervisor or HR representative about your return-to-work plan, including any adjustments to your schedule, workload, or responsibilities.

C. Negotiate Flexibility: Explore options for flexible work arrangements, such as telecommuting, flexible hours, or part-time schedules, to accommodate your needs as a working parent.

3. Prepare Emotionally:

A. Manage Expectations: Recognize that it's normal to experience a range of emotions as you prepare to return to work, including anxiety, guilt, and sadness. Be kind to yourself and acknowledge that it's okay to feel conflicted about leaving your baby.

B. Practice Self-Care: Prioritize self-care and stress management techniques, such as mindfulness, exercise, and relaxation, to support your emotional well-being during this challenging time.

C. Seek Support: Lean on your partner, family, and friends for emotional support and practical assistance as you navigate the transition back to work. Connect with other working parents for advice, encouragement, and solidarity.

4. Organize Work and Home:

A. Organize Workspace: Prepare your workspace for your return, organizing paperwork, setting up childcare arrangements, and ensuring you have everything you need to ease back into work smoothly.

B. Plan Transition: Develop a plan for transitioning your responsibilities back to work, including updating colleagues on project statuses, delegating tasks, and scheduling meetings to catch up on any developments during your absence.

C. Establish Routines: Establish routines and schedules for both work and home life to help you manage your time effectively and balance the demands of your professional and personal responsibilities.

5. Be Kind to Yourself:

A. Adjust Expectations: Recognize that it may take time to adjust to the demands of returning to work after maternity leave. Be patient with yourself and allow yourself grace as you navigate this transition.

B. Focus on Quality Time: Make the most of the time you have with your baby outside of work, focusing on quality over quantity and cherishing precious moments together.

C. Celebrate Achievements: Acknowledge and celebrate your achievements, both big and small, as you navigate the challenges of balancing work and family life. Give yourself credit for juggling multiple responsibilities and doing your best in each role.

Chapter 14: Pregnancy Complications

Common Issues: Gestational diabetes, preeclampsia, and other potential complications.

1. Gestational Diabetes:

A. Definition: Gestational diabetes mellitus (GDM) is a type of diabetes that develops during pregnancy, typically in the second or third trimester.

B. Risk Factors: Risk factors for gestational diabetes include being overweight or obese, having a family history of diabetes, being older than 25, or having had gestational diabetes in a previous pregnancy.

C. Symptoms: Gestational diabetes may not cause noticeable symptoms, but some women may experience increased thirst, frequent urination, fatigue, or blurred vision.

D. Complications: Untreated gestational diabetes can increase the risk of complications during pregnancy, including macrosomia (large birth weight), preterm birth, and cesarean delivery. It also raises the risk of developing type 2 diabetes later in life for both the mother and child.

E. Management: Treatment for gestational diabetes typically involves dietary modifications, regular exercise, blood glucose monitoring, and, in some cases, insulin therapy. Close monitoring by healthcare providers is essential to manage blood sugar levels and reduce the risk of complications.

2. Preeclampsia:

A. Definition: Preeclampsia is a pregnancy complication characterized by high blood pressure and signs of damage to organs, such as the liver and kidneys, after 20 weeks of pregnancy.

B. Risk Factors: Risk factors for preeclampsia include a history of preeclampsia in a previous pregnancy, first-time pregnancy, being older than 35, obesity, multiple gestation (twins or more), and certain medical conditions such as diabetes or kidney disease.

C. Symptoms: Symptoms of preeclampsia may include high blood pressure, protein in the urine, swelling (edema), headaches, vision changes, abdominal pain, and shortness of breath.

D. Complications: Preeclampsia can lead to serious complications for both the mother and baby, including eclampsia (seizures), HELLP syndrome (a combination of hemolysis, elevated liver enzymes, and low platelet count), placental abruption, preterm birth, and restricted fetal growth.

E. Management: Treatment for preeclampsia depends on the severity of the condition and how far along the pregnancy is. It may involve close monitoring of blood pressure and symptoms, bed rest, medication to lower blood pressure, and, in severe cases, early delivery of the baby to prevent complications.

3. Other Potential Complications:

A. Preterm Labor: Preterm labor, or labor that occurs before 37 weeks of pregnancy, can increase the risk of health problems for the baby, including respiratory distress syndrome, jaundice, and developmental delays.

B. Placenta Previa: Placenta previa occurs when the placenta partially or completely covers the cervix, increasing the risk of bleeding during pregnancy and delivery.

C. Miscarriage: Miscarriage, or the loss of a pregnancy before 20 weeks, is relatively common and can be caused by various factors, including chromosomal abnormalities, maternal age, and medical conditions.

D. Preterm Premature Rupture of Membranes (PPROM): PPROM occurs when the amniotic sac ruptures before 37 weeks of pregnancy, increasing the risk of infection and preterm delivery.

E. Intrauterine Growth Restriction (IUGR): IUGR refers to poor fetal growth and development, which can result from various factors, including maternal health conditions, placental problems, and genetic factors.

High-Risk Pregnancies: Special care and monitoring for high-risk pregnancies.

1. Factors Contributing to High-Risk Pregnancies:

A. Maternal Age: Women who are younger than 17 or older than 35 are considered at higher risk for complications due to increased likelihood of medical conditions and pregnancy-related issues.

B. Medical Conditions: Pre-existing medical conditions such as diabetes, hypertension, autoimmune disorders, heart disease, kidney disease, and certain infections can increase the risk of complications during pregnancy.

C. Multiple Gestations: Pregnancies with twins, triplets, or higher-order multiples are considered high-risk due to increased risks of preterm birth, low birth weight, and other complications.

D. Previous Pregnancy Complications: Women who have experienced pregnancy complications in previous pregnancies, such as preeclampsia, gestational diabetes, preterm birth, or stillbirth, are at increased risk of recurrence in subsequent pregnancies.

E. Lifestyle Factors: Smoking, alcohol consumption, drug use, obesity, and inadequate prenatal care can increase the risk of complications during pregnancy and childbirth.

2. Special Care and Monitoring:

A. Prenatal Care: High-risk pregnancies require close monitoring by healthcare providers, including more frequent prenatal visits and specialized tests or screenings to monitor the mother and baby's health.

B. Specialized Healthcare Providers: Women with high-risk pregnancies may be referred to maternal-fetal medicine specialists (perinatologists) or other healthcare providers with expertise in managing high-risk pregnancies.

C. Diagnostic Tests: Specialized diagnostic tests such as genetic screening, fetal ultrasound, Doppler flow studies, and fetal monitoring may be recommended to assess the baby's health and development and identify any potential complications.

D. Lifestyle Modifications: Women with high-risk pregnancies may be advised to make lifestyle modifications such as quitting smoking, avoiding alcohol and drugs, maintaining a healthy diet, and staying physically active under the guidance of a healthcare provider.

E. Medication and Treatment: Some women with high-risk pregnancies may require medication to manage medical conditions such as diabetes, hypertension, or autoimmune disorders. In severe cases, hospitalization or other medical interventions may be necessary to monitor and manage complications.

F. Psychosocial Support: High-risk pregnancies can be emotionally challenging for women and their families. Psychosocial support, counseling, and education can help women cope with stress, anxiety, and other emotional issues during pregnancy.

3. Birth Planning and Delivery:

A. Birth Plan: Women with high-risk pregnancies should develop a birth plan in consultation with their healthcare providers, outlining preferences for labor and delivery, pain management, and medical interventions.

B. Hospital Birth: Depending on the specific risk factors and complications, women with high-risk pregnancies may be advised to give birth in a hospital setting with access to specialized medical care and neonatal services.

C. Cesarean Delivery: In some cases, cesarean delivery (C-section) may be recommended to reduce the risk of complications for the mother or baby, such as in cases of placenta previa, fetal distress, or multiple gestations.

Chapter 15: Pregnancy After Loss

Coping with Loss: Emotional and physical recovery after miscarriage or stillbirth.

Emotional Recovery:

1. Allow Yourself to Grieve:

- Give yourself permission to feel and express your emotions, whether it's sadness, anger, guilt, or confusion. It's normal to experience a range of emotions after a loss, and it's essential to honor your feelings.

2. Seek Support:

- Lean on your partner, family, and friends for emotional support and comfort during this difficult time. Sharing your feelings and experiences with trusted loved ones can provide validation and help you feel less alone in your grief.

3. Join a Support Group:

- Consider joining a support group for individuals who have experienced pregnancy loss. Connecting with others who have gone through similar experiences can offer empathy, understanding, and a sense of community.

4. Express Yourself Creatively:

- Find healthy outlets for expressing your emotions, such as writing, journaling, drawing, painting, or creating art. Creative expression can be a therapeutic way to process grief and honor the memory of your lost pregnancy.

5. Practice Self-Compassion:

- Be gentle with yourself and practice self-compassion as you navigate the ups and downs of grief. Treat yourself with kindness, patience, and understanding, and recognize that healing takes time.

6. Consider Counseling or Therapy:

- If you're struggling to cope with your grief or finding it difficult to function in daily life, consider seeking professional counseling or therapy. A therapist trained in grief counseling can provide guidance, support, and coping strategies tailored to your needs.

Physical Recovery:

1. Rest and Recovery:

- Allow yourself time to rest and recover physically after a miscarriage or stillbirth. Listen to your body's cues and prioritize self-care activities such as getting enough sleep, eating nourishing foods, and avoiding strenuous activities.

2. Follow Medical Advice:

- Follow any medical advice or recommendations provided by your healthcare provider, including instructions for physical recovery, monitoring your health, and scheduling follow-up appointments.

3. Gentle Exercise:

- Engage in gentle exercise such as walking, yoga, or stretching to promote physical and emotional well-being. Exercise can help alleviate stress, improve mood, and support the body's healing process.

4. Monitor Symptoms:

- Pay attention to any physical symptoms or complications that may arise after a miscarriage or stillbirth, such as excessive bleeding, fever, pain, or signs of infection.

> Contact your healthcare provider if you have any concerns or questions about your physical recovery.

5. Be Patient with Your Body:

- Recognize that physical recovery takes time and varies from person to person. Be patient with your body as it heals and allow yourself grace as you navigate the physical aspects of grief and loss.

Trying Again: Preparing for another pregnancy after loss.

Emotional Preparation:

1. Allow Yourself to Heal:

- Give yourself permission to grieve and heal from the loss of your previous pregnancy. Take the time you need to process your emotions, honor your feelings, and work through any unresolved grief before trying to conceive again.

2. Communicate with Your Partner:

- Have open and honest conversations with your partner about your feelings, fears, and hopes for another pregnancy. Share your concerns and listen to each other's perspectives to strengthen your connection and support each other through the journey.

3. Seek Support:

- Lean on your support network of family, friends, and healthcare providers for emotional support and guidance as you navigate the decision to try for another pregnancy. Consider joining a support group for individuals who have experienced pregnancy loss to connect with others who understand your journey.

4. Address Anxiety and Fear:

- If you're experiencing anxiety or fear about trying for another pregnancy, consider seeking professional counseling or therapy to work through your feelings and develop coping strategies to manage anxiety and stress.

5. Practice Self-Care:

- Prioritize self-care activities that nurture your physical, emotional, and mental well-being, such as exercise, meditation, journaling, spending time in nature, or engaging in hobbies and activities you enjoy.

Practical Preparation:

1. Consult with Your Healthcare Provider:

- Schedule a preconception appointment with your healthcare provider to discuss your plans for another pregnancy and address any medical concerns or questions you may have. Your provider can offer guidance on optimizing your health and addressing any risk factors that may impact your fertility or pregnancy.

2. Address Medical Issues:

- If you have any underlying medical conditions that may affect fertility or pregnancy outcomes, work with your healthcare provider to manage these issues and optimize your health before trying to conceive again. This may include managing chronic health conditions, achieving a healthy weight, or addressing any fertility concerns.

3. Make Lifestyle Modifications:

- Adopt healthy lifestyle habits that support fertility and pregnancy, such as maintaining a balanced diet, exercising regularly, avoiding alcohol, tobacco, and illicit drugs, and managing stress effectively.

4. Monitor Ovulation and Fertility:

- Use ovulation tracking tools or methods to monitor your menstrual cycle and identify your most fertile days for conception. Consider using ovulation predictor kits, tracking basal body temperature, or monitoring cervical mucus changes to optimize timing for conception.

5. Prepare for Pregnancy:

- Take prenatal vitamins containing folic acid to support fetal development and reduce the risk of neural tube defects. Consider making any necessary preparations for pregnancy, such as updating your insurance coverage, creating a birth plan, or making arrangements for prenatal care.

Support Systems: Finding support groups and counseling.

Support Groups:

1. Online Resources:

- Explore online support groups and forums dedicated to pregnancy loss, infertility, and trying again. Websites, social media platforms, and online communities offer a wealth of resources and opportunities to connect with others who understand your experiences.

2. Local Organizations:

- Research local organizations, hospitals, or community centers that offer support groups or counseling services for individuals and couples coping with pregnancy loss or infertility. These groups may meet in person or virtually and provide a supportive environment for sharing stories, emotions, and coping strategies.

3. Healthcare Providers:

- Ask your healthcare provider for recommendations or referrals to support groups or counseling services specializing in pregnancy loss, infertility, or reproductive health. Many hospitals and clinics offer counseling services or can provide information about local support resources.

4. National Organizations:

- Reach out to national organizations dedicated to supporting individuals and families affected by pregnancy loss or infertility, such as the March of Dimes, Resolve: The National Infertility Association, or the Pregnancy Loss Support Program. These organizations may offer online resources, helplines, support groups, and educational materials.

5. Peer-Led Groups:

- Consider joining peer-led support groups facilitated by individuals who have personally experienced pregnancy loss or infertility. Peer support groups provide a unique opportunity to connect with others who share similar experiences and can offer empathy, validation, and practical advice based on firsthand knowledge.

Counseling:

1. Individual Counseling:

- Seek individual counseling or therapy with a licensed mental health professional specializing in pregnancy loss, infertility, or reproductive health. Counseling can provide a safe and confidential space to explore emotions, process grief, develop coping strategies, and work through any underlying issues contributing to distress.

2. Couples Counseling:

- Consider couples counseling or therapy with your partner to strengthen communication, navigate grief together, and address any relationship challenges or concerns related to pregnancy loss or infertility. Couples counseling can provide a supportive environment for processing emotions, fostering connection, and building resilience as a couple.

3. Fertility Counseling:

- If you're struggling with infertility or undergoing fertility treatments, consider seeking specialized fertility counseling or consultation with a reproductive psychologist or fertility counselor. Fertility counseling can provide emotional support, coping strategies, and decision-making guidance throughout the fertility journey.

4. Trauma-Informed Care:

- Look for counselors or therapists who have training and experience in trauma-informed care and understand the unique needs of individuals and couples affected by pregnancy loss or infertility. A trauma-informed approach emphasizes safety, trust, collaboration, and empowerment in the healing process.

5. Teletherapy Options:

- Explore teletherapy or online counseling options if in-person sessions are not feasible or accessible. Many therapists and counseling services offer virtual sessions via video conferencing or phone calls, allowing you to receive support from the comfort and convenience of your home.

Chapter 16: Special Conditions

Pregnancy Over 35: Risks and special care for older mothers.

Risks Associated with Pregnancy Over 35:

1. Fertility Decline:

- As women age, fertility gradually declines due to a decrease in the quantity and quality of eggs in the ovaries. This can increase the likelihood of infertility and difficulty conceiving naturally.

2. Increased Risk of Chromosomal Abnormalities:

- Advanced maternal age is associated with an increased risk of chromosomal abnormalities such as Down syndrome (trisomy 21) and other genetic disorders in the baby, primarily due to errors in egg production.

3. Higher Risk of Pregnancy Complications:

- Older mothers are at increased risk of pregnancy complications such as gestational diabetes, preeclampsia, placenta previa, placental abruption, preterm birth, and cesarean delivery.

4. Higher Likelihood of Multiple Gestation:

- The likelihood of conceiving twins or higher-order multiples increases with age, particularly with the use of assisted reproductive technologies (ART) such as in vitro fertilization (IVF).

5. Increased Risk of Stillbirth and Neonatal Death:

- Older maternal age is associated with a higher risk of stillbirth and neonatal death, although the absolute risk remains relatively low.

Special Care Recommendations for Older Mothers:

1. Preconception Counseling:

- If you're planning a pregnancy and are over 35, consider scheduling a preconception counseling appointment with your healthcare provider. Preconception counseling can help you understand the potential risks and make informed decisions about pregnancy timing and preparation.

2. Prenatal Genetic Counseling and Testing:

- Consider undergoing prenatal genetic counseling and testing, including noninvasive prenatal screening (NIPS) or diagnostic tests such as chorionic villus sampling (CVS) or amniocentesis, to assess the risk of chromosomal abnormalities and other genetic disorders in the baby.

3. Regular Prenatal Care:

- Attend regular prenatal care appointments with your healthcare provider to monitor your health and the baby's development closely. Prenatal care is essential for early detection and management of pregnancy complications and ensuring optimal maternal and fetal health.

4. Healthy Lifestyle Habits:

- Adopt healthy lifestyle habits to support a healthy pregnancy, including eating a balanced diet, maintaining a healthy weight, staying physically active (with guidance from your healthcare provider), avoiding alcohol, tobacco, and illicit drugs, and managing stress effectively.

5. Optimize Preexisting Health Conditions:

- If you have preexisting medical conditions such as diabetes, hypertension, or thyroid disorders, work with your healthcare provider to optimize your health before and during pregnancy. Proper management of chronic health conditions is crucial for reducing the risk of complications.

6. Discuss Birth Planning and Delivery Options:

- Discuss birth planning and delivery options with your healthcare provider, including considerations for labor induction, cesarean delivery, and postpartum care. Be prepared to discuss your preferences and concerns regarding childbirth and postpartum recovery.

7. Consideration for Assisted Reproductive Technologies (ART):

- If you're experiencing infertility or difficulty conceiving, consider consulting a fertility specialist to explore options for assisted reproductive technologies (ART) such as IVF or intrauterine insemination (IUI) to improve your chances of conceiving.

Chronic Conditions: Managing pregnancy with diabetes, hypertension, or other chronic illnesses.

1. Preconception Planning:

A. Preconception Counseling:

- If you have a chronic condition and are planning a pregnancy, schedule a preconception counseling appointment with your healthcare provider. Preconception counseling can help you understand how your condition may affect pregnancy and develop a plan to optimize your health before conception.

B. Medication Review:

- Review your current medications with your healthcare provider to ensure they are safe to continue during pregnancy. Some medications may need to be adjusted or changed to minimize risks to the baby.

C. Achieve Optimal Health:

- Work with your healthcare provider to achieve optimal health before pregnancy by managing your chronic condition effectively, maintaining a healthy weight, eating a balanced diet, exercising regularly, and avoiding harmful substances.

2. Prenatal Care:

A. Regular Prenatal Visits:

- Attend regular prenatal care appointments with your healthcare provider to monitor your health and the baby's development closely. Prenatal visits are essential for early detection and management of complications related to your chronic condition.

B. Blood Pressure Monitoring:

- If you have hypertension or other cardiovascular conditions, monitor your blood pressure regularly at home and report any high readings to your healthcare provider. Proper blood pressure control is crucial for reducing the risk of complications such as preeclampsia.

C. Blood Glucose Monitoring:

- If you have diabetes or gestational diabetes, monitor your blood glucose levels regularly and follow your healthcare provider's recommendations for insulin or medication management, diet, and exercise. Tight glycemic control is essential for reducing the risk of complications for both mother and baby.

3. Lifestyle Modifications:

A. Healthy Diet:

- Follow a balanced diet rich in fruits, vegetables, whole grains, lean proteins, and healthy fats to support optimal maternal and fetal health. Limiting processed foods, sugary snacks, and excessive salt intake can help manage chronic conditions such as diabetes and hypertension.

B. Regular Exercise:

- Engage in regular physical activity under the guidance of your healthcare provider. Exercise can help control blood sugar levels, lower blood pressure, improve circulation, and reduce stress during pregnancy.

C. Stress Management:

- Practice stress-reducing techniques such as deep breathing, meditation, yoga, or mindfulness to manage stress and promote emotional well-being during pregnancy.

4. Medication Management:

A. Compliance with Medications:

- Take your medications as prescribed by your healthcare provider and follow their recommendations for dosage adjustments or changes during pregnancy.

B. Potential Risks and Benefits:

- Discuss the potential risks and benefits of medications with your healthcare provider to make informed decisions about treatment options that are safe and effective for managing your chronic condition during pregnancy.

5. Communication and Collaboration:

A. Open Communication:

- Maintain open and honest communication with your healthcare provider about any concerns, symptoms, or changes in your health during pregnancy. Your healthcare provider can offer guidance, support, and adjustments to your treatment plan as needed.

B. Collaboration with Specialists:

- Depending on the complexity of your chronic condition, you may need to collaborate with specialists such as endocrinologists, cardiologists, or obstetricians who have expertise in managing high-risk pregnancies.

Lifestyle Considerations: Adjustments for a healthy pregnancy with existing health conditions.

1. Balanced Diet:

A. Nutrient-Rich Foods:

- Focus on consuming a balanced diet rich in fruits, vegetables, whole grains, lean proteins, and healthy fats. Aim to include a variety of nutrient-dense foods to support optimal maternal and fetal health.

B. Blood Sugar Management:

- If you have diabetes or gestational diabetes, monitor your carbohydrate intake and distribute it evenly throughout the day to help stabilize blood sugar levels. Limit sugary snacks and beverages and opt for complex carbohydrates with high fiber content.

C. Sodium Intake:

- If you have hypertension or cardiovascular conditions, limit your sodium intake by reducing processed foods, canned soups, salty snacks, and fast food. Opt for fresh, whole foods and use herbs and spices to flavor meals instead of salt.

2. Regular Exercise:

A. Safe Physical Activity:

- Engage in regular physical activity under the guidance of your healthcare provider. Choose low-impact exercises such as walking, swimming, prenatal yoga, or stationary cycling to promote cardiovascular health, strengthen muscles, and improve overall well-being.

B. Blood Sugar Control:

- Physical activity can help regulate blood sugar levels in women with diabetes or gestational diabetes. Aim for at least 30 minutes of moderate-intensity exercise most days of the week, and monitor blood sugar levels before and after exercise.

3. Weight Management:

A. Healthy Weight Gain:

- Aim for appropriate weight gain during pregnancy based on recommendations from your healthcare provider. Excessive weight gain can exacerbate health conditions such as diabetes and hypertension, while inadequate weight gain may increase the risk of complications for the baby.

B. Nutrition Counseling:

- Consider seeking guidance from a registered dietitian or nutritionist specializing in pregnancy and chronic conditions. A nutritionist can help you develop a personalized meal plan and make dietary adjustments to support your health and the baby's development.

4. Stress Management:

A. Relaxation Techniques:

- Practice stress-reducing techniques such as deep breathing, meditation, mindfulness, progressive muscle relaxation, or guided imagery to manage stress and promote emotional well-being during pregnancy.

B. Support Systems:

- Lean on your support network of family, friends, and healthcare providers for emotional support and practical assistance. Consider joining support groups or seeking counseling to connect with others who understand your experiences.

5. Medication Management:

A. Compliance with Medications:

- Take your medications as prescribed by your healthcare provider and follow their recommendations for dosage adjustments or changes during pregnancy. Do not stop or adjust medications without consulting your healthcare provider.

B. Medication Safety:

- Discuss the safety of medications with your healthcare provider, especially if you have concerns about potential risks to the baby. Your healthcare provider can help you weigh the benefits and risks of medication use during pregnancy and make informed decisions about treatment options.

6. Regular Prenatal Care:

A. Monitoring Health:

- Attend regular prenatal care appointments with your healthcare provider to monitor your health and the baby's development closely. Prenatal visits are essential for early detection and management of complications related to your health condition.

B. Communication with Healthcare Provider:

- Maintain open and honest communication with your healthcare provider about any concerns, symptoms, or changes in your health during pregnancy. Your healthcare provider can offer guidance, support, and adjustments to your treatment plan as needed.

Chapter 17: Partner's Role

Supportive Partner: How partners can support the pregnant mother.

Emotional Support:

1. **Active Listening:**
   o Take the time to listen attentively to the pregnant mother's thoughts, feelings, and concerns without judgment. Offer empathy, understanding, and validation of her experiences.
2. **Encouragement and Affirmation:**
   o Offer words of encouragement, praise, and affirmation to boost the pregnant mother's confidence and morale. Remind her of her strength, resilience, and capabilities as she navigates the challenges of pregnancy.
3. **Validation of Emotions:**

o   Validate the pregnant mother's emotions and experiences, acknowledging that pregnancy can bring a wide range of feelings, including joy, anxiety, fear, and uncertainty. Let her know that it's okay to feel whatever she's feeling.

4. **Participation in Prenatal Activities:**

o   Attend prenatal appointments, ultrasound scans, and childbirth education classes with the pregnant mother to show your support and involvement in her pregnancy journey. Ask questions, engage with healthcare providers, and be present during important milestones.

Physical Support:

1. **Assistance with Household Tasks:**

o   Help with household chores, errands, and responsibilities to alleviate the pregnant mother's physical burden and fatigue. Offer to cook meals, do laundry, clean the house, and run errands as needed.

2. **Physical Comfort Measures:**

o   Offer physical comfort measures such as back rubs, foot massages, and warm baths to help relieve pregnancy-related aches, pains, and discomforts. Provide pillows for support during sleep and encourage rest and relaxation.

3. **Accommodations for Comfort:**

o   Make accommodations to ensure the pregnant mother's comfort and well-being, such as adjusting the thermostat to a comfortable temperature, providing extra pillows for support, and creating a relaxing environment at home.

4. **Assistance with Mobility:**

o   Offer assistance with mobility, especially as the pregnancy progresses and the pregnant mother may experience limitations in movement. Help her with tasks such as getting in and out of bed, standing up, and moving around safely.

Practical Support:

1. **Financial Planning and Preparation:**
   - Work together to create a budget, plan for baby-related expenses, and make financial preparations for the arrival of the baby. Discuss parental leave, healthcare costs, childcare options, and other practical considerations.
2. **Baby-Related Tasks and Preparations:**
   - Assist with baby-related tasks and preparations, such as setting up the nursery, assembling baby gear, and purchasing essential items for the baby's arrival. Take an active role in preparing for parenthood together.
3. **Research and Education:**
   - Conduct research and educate yourselves about pregnancy, childbirth, and parenting topics. Attend childbirth education classes, read books, and seek reliable information to prepare for the journey ahead as parents.
4. **Flexibility and Adaptability:**
   - Be flexible and adaptable in your roles and responsibilities, recognizing that pregnancy and parenthood may require adjustments and compromises. Communicate openly and collaboratively to find solutions that work for both of you.

Communication and Partnership:

1. **Open Communication:**
   - Foster open, honest, and respectful communication with the pregnant mother, sharing your thoughts, feelings, and concerns openly. Keep the lines of communication open

and address any issues or challenges together as a team.

2. **Shared Decision-Making:**
   - Involve the pregnant mother in decision-making processes related to pregnancy, childbirth, and parenting. Respect her preferences, values, and choices, and collaborate on important decisions that impact both of you and the baby.

3. **Mutual Support and Encouragement:**
   - Offer mutual support and encouragement to each other as partners, acknowledging that pregnancy and parenthood are shared experiences that require teamwork, patience, and mutual understanding. Celebrate achievements and milestones together.

Involvement: Ways for partners to be involved in the pregnancy and birth process.

During Pregnancy:

1. **Attend Prenatal Appointments:**
   - Accompany the pregnant mother to prenatal appointments, ultrasounds, and check-ups whenever possible. Ask questions, engage with healthcare providers, and be an active participant in discussions about the pregnancy.

2. **Educate Yourself:**
   - Take the time to educate yourself about pregnancy, childbirth, and parenting. Read books, attend childbirth education classes, and seek reliable information to better understand the pregnancy journey and prepare for parenthood.

3. **Support Healthy Lifestyle Habits:**
   - Encourage and support the pregnant mother in maintaining healthy lifestyle habits, such as eating a balanced diet, staying physically active, getting enough rest, and managing stress.

Offer to join her in exercise activities and prepare nutritious meals together.

4. **Provide Emotional Support:**
o   Offer emotional support and encouragement to the pregnant mother throughout the pregnancy. Listen attentively to her thoughts and feelings, validate her experiences, and reassure her of your love and support.

5. **Bond with the Baby:**
o   Take proactive steps to bond with the baby during pregnancy, such as talking, singing, and reading to the baby bump. Attend childbirth education classes together to learn about labor, birth, and newborn care.

6. **Prepare for Parenthood:**
o   Work together to prepare for parenthood by discussing parenting styles, values, and expectations. Attend parenting workshops or support groups to learn practical skills and strategies for caring for a newborn.

During Labor and Birth:

1. **Be the Birth Partner:**
o   Serve as the primary birth partner and advocate for the pregnant mother during labor and birth. Provide physical comfort measures, emotional support, and reassurance throughout the birthing process.

2. **Attend Childbirth Classes:**
o   Attend childbirth education classes with the pregnant mother to learn about labor stages, comfort techniques, and pain management options. Practice relaxation techniques and labor positions together.

3. **Assist with Labor Support:**
o   Assist the pregnant mother with breathing exercises, massage, positioning, and other comfort measures during labor. Offer words of encouragement and reassurance to help her stay focused and empowered.

4. **Communicate with Healthcare Providers:**

o   Communicate the pregnant mother's preferences, concerns, and birth plan to healthcare providers during labor. Advocate for her needs and wishes while respecting medical advice and recommendations.

5. **Capture Memories:**

o   Take photos or videos to capture special moments during labor and birth, with the pregnant mother's consent. Document the journey and celebrate the arrival of your baby together as a family.

After Birth:

1.   **Provide Postpartum Support:**

o   Offer emotional support, practical assistance, and encouragement to the new mother during the postpartum period. Help with newborn care tasks, household chores, and errands to ease her transition into motherhood.

2.   **Bond with the Baby:**

o   Take an active role in bonding with the baby by participating in feeding, diaper changes, bathing, and soothing activities. Spend quality time together as a family and create lasting memories with your newborn.

3.   **Support Breastfeeding:**

o   Support the new mother in her breastfeeding journey by providing encouragement, assistance with positioning and latch, and practical support. Offer to help with burping, diaper changes, and other tasks to facilitate breastfeeding success.

4.   **Share Responsibilities:**

o   Share parenting responsibilities and household tasks equitably with your partner. Collaborate on caregiving duties, decision-making, and scheduling to ensure both parents feel supported and involved in parenting.

5.   **Celebrate Milestones:**

  o Celebrate milestones and achievements together as a family, such as the baby's first smile, first steps, and other developmental milestones. Cherish these special moments and create a supportive and nurturing environment for your growing family.

Emotional Support: Helping partners cope with their own feelings and stress.

1. Encourage Open Communication:

1. **Create a Safe Space:** Foster an environment of trust and openness where partners feel comfortable expressing their thoughts, feelings, and concerns without judgment or criticism.
2. **Active Listening:** Practice active listening by giving partners your full attention, maintaining eye contact, and offering empathy and validation of their experiences.
3. **Ask Open-Ended Questions:** Encourage partners to share their feelings and thoughts by asking open-ended questions that invite deeper conversation and reflection.

2. Validate Their Emotions:

1. **Acknowledge Feelings:** Validate partners' emotions by acknowledging and accepting their feelings without trying to dismiss or minimize them.
2. **Normalize Emotions:** Remind partners that it's normal to experience a range of emotions during pregnancy and parenthood, including anxiety, fear, excitement, and uncertainty.
3. **Provide Reassurance:** Offer reassurance and encouragement to partners, reminding them that they are not alone and that their feelings are valid and understandable.

3. Offer Practical Support:

1. **Share Responsibilities:** Share household tasks, childcare duties, and other responsibilities to alleviate partners' stress and workload. Collaborate on caregiving tasks and decision-making to ensure both partners feel supported and valued.
2. **Take Breaks:** Encourage partners to take breaks and engage in self-care activities to recharge and replenish their energy. Offer to watch the baby or handle household chores while they take time for themselves.
3. **Provide Physical Comfort:** Offer physical comfort measures such as hugs, cuddles, and affectionate gestures to reassure partners of your love and support.

4. Seek Professional Help if Needed:

1. **Normalize Therapy:** Normalize the idea of seeking professional help if partners are struggling with overwhelming emotions or stress. Offer support and encouragement to attend therapy or counseling sessions to address their mental health needs.
2. **Connect with Support Groups:** Encourage partners to connect with other parents or support groups where they can share their experiences, gain perspective, and receive empathy and understanding from others who can relate to their struggles.
3. **Offer to Accompany:** Offer to accompany partners to therapy sessions or support group meetings if they feel apprehensive or hesitant about attending alone. Provide reassurance and

encouragement to take proactive steps towards self-care and emotional well-being.

5. Be Patient and Understanding:

1. **Practice Patience:** Be patient and understanding with partners as they navigate their own emotions and stressors. Offer unconditional support and reassurance, even if you may not fully understand or relate to their experiences.
2. **Validate Their Experience:** Validate partners' experiences and feelings, even if they may differ from your own. Respect their perspective and acknowledge the unique challenges they may be facing.
3. **Show Gratitude:** Express gratitude for partners' efforts and contributions to the relationship and family. Acknowledge their support and sacrifices, and let them know that their well-being is important to you.

Education and Resources: Books, classes, and resources for new parents.

Books for New Parents:

1. **"What to Expect When You're Expecting" by Heidi Murkoff and Sharon Mazel:**
   o This comprehensive guide covers everything from conception to childbirth, providing practical advice, tips, and information on pregnancy, labor, and delivery.
2. **"The Expectant Father" by Armin A. Brott and Jennifer Ash:**

- o Geared towards expectant fathers, this book offers insights, guidance, and advice on how to support your partner during pregnancy, childbirth, and the early stages of fatherhood.
3. **"The Baby Book: Everything You Need to Know About Your Baby from Birth to Age Two" by William Sears, Martha Sears, and Robert Sears:**
- o Written by renowned pediatricians, this book covers all aspects of baby care, including breastfeeding, sleep, nutrition, and development, providing evidence-based information and practical tips for new parents.
4. **"Bringing Up Bébé: One American Mother Discovers the Wisdom of French Parenting" by Pamela Druckerman:**
- o This book explores the differences in parenting styles between American and French cultures, offering insights and lessons on raising children with confidence, independence, and resilience.
5. **"The Happiest Baby on the Block" by Harvey Karp:**
- o Dr. Harvey Karp shares his techniques for soothing and calming newborns, offering practical strategies for parents to help their babies sleep better and cry less.

Childbirth Education Classes:

1. **Childbirth Preparation Classes:**
- o Many hospitals and birthing centers offer childbirth preparation classes for expectant parents. These classes cover topics such as labor and delivery, pain management techniques, relaxation exercises, breastfeeding, and newborn care.
2. **Breastfeeding Classes:**
- o Breastfeeding classes provide expectant parents with information, guidance, and support for successful breastfeeding. They cover topics such as latching, positioning, milk supply, pumping, and troubleshooting common breastfeeding challenges.
3. **Newborn Care Classes:**

o   Newborn care classes focus on essential skills and knowledge for caring for a newborn, including diapering, bathing, soothing techniques, sleep safety, and recognizing signs of illness or distress.

4. **Parenting Workshops and Support Groups:**

o   Consider attending parenting workshops and support groups in your community or online. These groups offer opportunities to connect with other parents, share experiences, and gain insights and advice from experts and experienced caregivers.

Online Resources:

1.   **American Pregnancy Association (APA):**

o   The APA website offers a wealth of information on pregnancy, childbirth, and parenting, including articles, videos, FAQs, and resources on various topics related to pregnancy and parenthood.

2.   **BabyCenter:**

o   BabyCenter provides information and resources for expectant and new parents, including articles, expert advice, community forums, and tools such as pregnancy trackers and baby name finders.

3.   **La Leche League International (LLLI):**

o   LLLI offers evidence-based information and support for breastfeeding mothers, including online resources, articles, forums, and local support groups led by trained breastfeeding counselors.

4.   **Postpartum Support International (PSI):**

o   PSI offers support and resources for new parents dealing with postpartum mood disorders such as postpartum depression and anxiety. Their website provides information, helplines, and resources for finding support and treatment options.

5.   **Centers for Disease Control and Prevention (CDC):**

- o The CDC website offers resources and guidelines on various aspects of pregnancy, childbirth, and newborn care, including prenatal care, breastfeeding, vaccination, and infant health and development.

Chapter 18: Reflecting on the Journey

Looking Back: Reflecting on the highs and lows of your pregnancy journey.

Highs:

1. **Joy of Discovery:** The journey began with the joyous discovery of pregnancy, a moment filled with excitement, anticipation, and dreams of the future.
2. **Bonding with Baby:** As the pregnancy progressed, there were countless moments of bonding with the baby, from feeling the first fluttering kicks to seeing the baby's ultrasound images for the first time.
3. **Supportive Network:** Surrounding ourselves with a supportive network of family, friends, and healthcare providers was a constant source of strength and encouragement throughout the journey.
4. **Milestone Moments:** Celebrating milestone moments such as gender reveal parties, baby showers, and prenatal appointments filled us with happiness and gratitude for the blessing of new life.
5. **Nesting and Preparation:** The process of nesting and preparing for the baby's arrival brought a sense of purpose and excitement, from decorating the nursery to assembling baby gear and creating birth plans.
6. **Shared Journey:** Sharing the pregnancy journey with my partner deepened our bond and strengthened our relationship, as we navigated the highs and lows together with love, support, and understanding.

Lows:

1. **Physical Discomfort:** Coping with physical discomforts such as morning sickness, fatigue, and back pain was challenging at times, requiring patience, self-care, and resilience.
2. **Emotional Rollercoaster:** The emotional ups and downs of pregnancy, including mood swings, anxiety, and uncertainty, tested our emotional resilience and required us to lean on each other for support.
3. **Health Concerns:** Dealing with health concerns or complications during pregnancy, such as gestational diabetes or high blood pressure, added stress and anxiety to the journey, requiring close monitoring and medical intervention.
4. **Uncertainty and Anxiety:** The uncertainty of the future and worries about childbirth, parenting, and the well-being of the baby sometimes kept us awake at night, reminding us of the weight of responsibility that comes with parenthood.
5. **Navigating Changes:** Adjusting to the physical, emotional, and lifestyle changes that come with pregnancy required flexibility, adaptability, and self-care to maintain balance and well-being.
6. **Unexpected Challenges:** Facing unexpected challenges or setbacks along the way, such as pregnancy complications or unexpected changes in birth plans, tested our resilience and forced us to confront fears and uncertainties head-on.

Personal Growth: Recognizing the personal growth and changes you've experienced.

Self-awareness and Resilience:

1. **Increased Self-awareness:** Throughout the pregnancy journey, I developed a deeper understanding of myself, my strengths, and my limitations. Facing challenges and uncertainties allowed me to explore my emotions, values, and priorities, leading to greater self-awareness and self-discovery.
2. **Enhanced Resilience:** Coping with the physical discomforts, emotional ups and downs, and unexpected challenges of pregnancy fostered resilience within me. I learned to adapt to change, overcome obstacles, and bounce back from setbacks with determination and perseverance.

Emotional Intelligence and Empathy:

1. **Heightened Emotional Intelligence:** Navigating the emotional rollercoaster of pregnancy heightened my emotional intelligence, enabling me to recognize and manage my own emotions more effectively. I became more attuned to the emotions of others, fostering deeper connections and empathy in my relationships.
2. **Increased Empathy:** Experiencing the highs and lows of pregnancy deepened my empathy for others going through similar experiences. I gained a greater appreciation for the challenges faced by expectant parents and developed a more compassionate outlook towards those in need of support.

Strengthened Relationships:

1. **Deeper Connection with Partner:** Sharing the pregnancy journey with my partner strengthened our bond and deepened our connection as we navigated the joys and challenges together. We learned to communicate more openly, support each other unconditionally, and face adversity as a united team.
2. **Enhanced Family Dynamics:** The pregnancy journey also had a profound impact on my relationships with family members and loved ones. We rallied together to celebrate milestones, offer encouragement, and create a supportive network of love and solidarity.

Heightened Sense of Responsibility:

1. **Parental Instincts:** As the pregnancy progressed, I experienced a growing sense of responsibility and readiness to embrace the role of a parent. I felt a deepening connection with the unborn baby, nurturing feelings of love, protection, and devotion.
2. **Commitment to Parenting:** The anticipation of becoming a parent fueled my commitment to providing a nurturing and loving environment for the baby. I became more proactive in educating myself about childcare, parenting techniques, and fostering a positive family environment.

Gratitude and Appreciation:

1. **Gratitude for the Miracle of Life:** Throughout the pregnancy journey, I cultivated a profound sense of gratitude for the miracle of life and the privilege of becoming a parent. I cherished each moment, from feeling the baby's kicks to witnessing the growth and development during ultrasounds.
2. **Appreciation for Support:** I am grateful for the unwavering support of my partner, family, friends, and healthcare providers who stood by me every step of the way. Their encouragement, guidance, and love have been invaluable in shaping my journey towards parenthood.

Moving Forward: Preparing for the next chapter of parenthood and embracing the future.

1. Final Preparations:

1. **Nesting and Baby-proofing:** Complete any remaining preparations for the baby's arrival, including nesting activities like organizing the nursery, assembling baby furniture, and baby-proofing the home.
2. **Gathering Essentials:** Ensure you have all the necessary baby essentials such as diapers, clothing, feeding supplies, and baby gear ready for when the baby arrives.
3. **Creating a Birth Plan:** Finalize your birth plan with your healthcare provider, outlining your preferences for labor, delivery, and postpartum care. Be prepared to be flexible and adapt to any changes that may arise during labor and birth.

2. Self-care and Well-being:

1. **Prioritizing Self-care:** Make self-care a priority as you prepare for parenthood. Engage in activities that promote relaxation, stress relief, and well-being, such as meditation, yoga, exercise, and spending time outdoors.
2. **Seeking Support:** Lean on your support network of family, friends, and healthcare providers for emotional support and practical assistance as needed. Don't hesitate to reach out for help or guidance when you need it.
3. **Communicating with Your Partner:** Maintain open and honest communication with your partner as you navigate the transition to parenthood together. Share your thoughts, feelings, and concerns, and work together as a team to support each other.

3. Educating Yourself:

1. **Parenting Resources:** Continue educating yourself about parenting techniques, newborn care, breastfeeding, and child development. Take advantage of books, classes, online resources, and support groups to enhance your knowledge and skills as a parent.
2. **Preparing for Challenges:** Recognize that parenthood comes with its own set of challenges and uncertainties. Prepare yourself mentally and emotionally to navigate the ups and downs of parenting with patience, resilience, and flexibility.
3. **Learning from Others:** Seek advice and guidance from experienced parents who can offer insights, tips, and encouragement based on their own experiences. Remember that every parent and baby is unique, so trust your instincts and do what feels right for your family.

4. Embracing the Future:

1. **Cultivating Joy and Anticipation:** Embrace the future with a sense of joy, anticipation, and excitement for the journey ahead. Focus on the positive aspects of parenthood and look forward to creating cherished memories with your growing family.
2. **Embracing Parenthood:** Embrace the role of parenthood with an open heart and a willingness to learn and grow along the way. Embrace the challenges, triumphs, and everyday moments that come with raising a child, knowing that each experience contributes to the richness of family life.
3. **Creating Memories:** Cherish each moment with your baby and create lasting memories as you embark on the adventure of parenthood together. Take time to savor the small joys, celebrate milestones, and nurture the bond between parent and child.

Conclusion:

As we conclude our exploration of "The Pregnancy Blueprint," we are filled with gratitude for the opportunity to embark on this journey together. We have shared in the joys and challenges of pregnancy, celebrated the miracle of new life, and prepared for the adventure of parenthood with open hearts and eager anticipation. As we look ahead to the future, we are reminded that the journey of parenthood is not without its obstacles, but with love, support, and determination, we can overcome any challenge and embrace the joys of raising a child. Thank you for joining us on this transformative journey, and may your path to parenthood be filled with love, happiness, and countless blessings.

www.ingramcontent.com/pod-product-compliance
Lightning Source LLC
Chambersburg PA
CBHW061634250726
48659CB00004B/1219